Bedtime
Stories
to Help You
Sleep

Just Sleep

PRESENTS

Bedtime Stories to Help You Sleep

RELAXING TALES FOR ADULTS

EDITED BY

Taesha Glasgow

ASTER*

First published in Great Britain in 2025 by Aster, an imprint of
Octopus Publishing Group Ltd
Carmelite House
50 Victoria Embankment
London EC4Y 0DZ
www.octopusbooks.co.uk

An Hachette UK Company
www.hachette.co.uk

The authorized representative in the EEA is Hachette Ireland,
8 Castlecourt Centre, Dublin 15, D15 XTP3, Ireland (email: info@hbgi.ie)

Introduction copyright © Taesha Glasgow, 2025

Distributed in the US by Hachette Book Group
1290 Avenue of the Americas, 4th and 5th Floors
New York, NY 10104

Distributed in Canada by Canadian Manda Group
664 Annette St., Toronto, Ontario, Canada M6S 2C8

ISBN (hardback): 978-1-78325-658-7
ISBN (trade paperback): 978-1-78325-660-0
eISBN: 978-1-78325-659-4

A CIP catalogue record for this book is available from the British Library.

Typeset in 11/15pt Sabon LT Pro Six Red Marbles, Thetford, Norfolk

Printed and bound in Great Britain

1 3 5 7 9 10 8 6 4 2

Commissioning editor: Jessica Minocha
Senior developmental editor: Pauline Bache
Copyeditor: Ian Critchley
Creative director: Mel Four
Production controller: Sarah Parry

'Beauty and the Beast' translated by James Planche
'Verotchka' translated by Constance Garnett

This FSC® label means that materials used for the product have been responsibly sourced.

To Paul. The show would not have been possible without you. We make a great team. Love you.

CONTENTS

INTRODUCTION

I have a confession to make. It takes me minutes to fall asleep. Sometimes seconds. I have been known to fall asleep mid-sentence, holding a book I'm reading or sitting upright in a chair. But my husband is the complete opposite. He could take hours to fall asleep. Often waking up in the night and not being able to settle back down to rest, thinking about the day ahead or mulling over the previous day's challenges. It had always been this way. Then the pandemic happened and everything got worse. My consulting business was nosediving, stress and anxiety were up, as were unpaid bills. We tried to stay positive and juggle everything around (like most people on the planet at that time), then my husband, Paul, fell ill suddenly.

After this, a good night's sleep became even more essential. The playlists and YouTube videos weren't cutting it. One night, while he was selecting a *Fall of Civilizations* episode on YouTube, I casually suggested that maybe I should read to him to help him sleep. We laughed for a moment but the laughter ended with a question mark. Would this help him? Were there other people struggling at that time that we could help too?

Four months of research and numerous test recordings later, we launched the podcast *Just Sleep: Bedtime Stories for Adults*. The positive response was immediate and exceeded our reasonable expectations. Within weeks, we received messages from listeners stating that the show was helping them calm their restless minds at the end of the day. They listened to the stories with their children and the show helped to make bedtimes more special. The show helped them so much that they were able to ease off their sleep medication. Now, over three hundred episodes and almost twenty million downloads later, we still get messages like those from our listeners and it drives us to continue to produce the show, two episodes per week.

The decision to create this book was easy. We want to continue our mission to help more people relax, put the stressful day behind them and drift off to sleep. Some of the stories in this book are from the most popular episodes on the podcast. Not only the episodes with the most downloads, but stories that listeners have told us time and time again that they love and listen to over and over again. Like the timeless fairytale 'Beauty and the Beast', the chapter filled with wonder from *The Wind in the Willows* and some Sherlock Holmes mysteries (our listeners love Sherlock Holmes so much, I included him twice in this collection). More stories are exclusive to this book. I have selected classics from Katherine Mansfield, Anton Chekhov and Maurice Leblanc; perfect if you want a story that simply soothes you or if you want a tale with a little more bite. I hope you love these stories as much as I loved selecting them for you. Goodnight.

THE WOMAN WHO WAS SO TIRED

Elizabeth Banks

The assistant editor wanted a story with 'human interest' in it, so he looked around for the Little Reporter.

She came whirling in on the wings of the revolving door, dancing on her toes to keep up a circulation, her fingers wiggling within her muff, her veil dotted with frozen tear drops.

'My! It's cold!' she piped, 'and so glassy, I slipped twice getting here from the elevated.'

Throwing her frosted muff and coat on her roll-top desk she lovingly hugged the radiator, holding in her half-numbed fingers the morning paper, while she scanned the headlines.

They called her 'the Little Reporter' because she was no bigger than your thumb and because she belonged to that particular type of woman which always appeals to the male heart as needing to be taken care of.

'Yes,' said the assistant editor, 'it is cold, and the weather has made me think of a story for you. New York must be full of suffering of one kind and another on a day like this. Just go out and spend it looking for the coldest woman in New York, or the saddest woman, or the most overworked woman, or the most anything woman in New York, and come back and write a story about her.'

So the Little Reporter drew on her coat and dried her veil and wrapped it about her face, and skipped blithely out by the circling door into the sleet, and late that night she came back and sat at her desk and wrote a story, and she called it 'The Woman Who Was So Tired'.

While the assistant editor read the copy it was noticed that he used his handkerchief freely, while swearing at whoever it might be who insisted upon having fresh air from an open window.

'And me coming down with this cold in my head!' muttered the assistant editor unsteadily.

The story of 'The Woman Who Was So Tired' made a hit. It was full of humour and a tender pathos that touched the heart. In it the Little Reporter seemed to have given her readers of her best, that best which made the smile break through the tears like a sunburst through an April shower. People read, and as they read they laughed with 'The Woman Who Was So Tired' at the comedies in her daily life, while as quickly they wept over her tragedies.

'The Woman Who Was So Tired' was described as young and self-supporting, and others-supporting as well, for she had a mother who stopped at home and kept the flat between the intervals of pain; two little sisters in the graded school and a young brother.

To earn their several livings 'The Woman Who Was So Tired' had chosen a profession which made of her a wanderer in New York's streets, among the rich, the poor, the moderately well-to-do. Did not one know without a telling that she was a book canvasser or a seller of small wares at open doors – doors that so often shut in her face ere she had stated her errand?

All day she wandered among downtown offices, east side tenements, west side apartments. Sometimes into shops on Fifth Avenue and Broadway, sometimes into those of humble, dirty side streets; sometimes she searched for treasure among the garbage cans. There were days when, in connection with her own legitimate business, she would attempt to aid those who were in greater distress than herself, and on certain of these days there were high-pitched voices that assailed her and brooms held in filthy hands would almost sweep her down a squalid five flights of stairs. The longer she worked the better she was likely to be paid, for she worked on a pitiful commission.

Often when in the worst neighbourhoods of the east side she would go hungry all the day, not always because she lacked the pennies for food, but because her capricious appetite revolted against the fare served in any of the nearby restaurants.

She was often running to catch cars and trains, for minutes were precious to her; and she sometimes walked, seeking out her patrons, so she was always weary, and in writing of her the Little Reporter had named her 'The Woman Who Was So Tired'.

At the newspaper office they knew at once the story had made a hit, because it brought in letters by the dozens. Kind-hearted philanthropists demanded to be given the real name and address of 'The Woman Who Was So Tired', for they knew she lived and moved among them every day and that the author of the story had met her and known her well. She had gone to their hearts and they wanted to do something for her. One saw that the weary woman was proud, though poor, so the philanthropists declared they would help her without her knowing whence help came. Working women wrote, thanking the author for her championship of women who had to work overtime, for the heroine had been described as often working sixteen hours a day.

Before the end of the week the volume of correspondence concerning the story and its heroine so increased that now the Little Reporter had it heaped upon her desk in stacks, and presents began to arrive addressed to 'The Woman Who Was So Tired' in care of the editor or the writer of the story. Cheques came in, and the Little Reporter gashed the palm of her hand with pins that fastened dollar bills to note paper on which was daintily written or ignorantly scrawled a word of sympathy for the heroine of roving feet.

There were presents of warm clothing, dress lengths, toys of various kinds for the little sisters and brother, a thin Coalport cup and saucer for the invalid mother who in the story longed for the dainty surroundings of better days; there were books, some grave, some laughter-giving, all nicely bound; boxes of chocolates, packages of nuts.

Very frequently the assistant editor would be called to the telephone to be asked for the address or further information of 'The Woman Who Was So Tired', and he grew irritable over the continual interruptions to his work. 'One might think,' he said crossly, 'that nobody ever was tired before and never would be again. Great Scott! I'm tired myself. Here!' he called to Bobbie, the office boy, 'take this batch of letters and presents over to Miss Sanderson's desk and tell her to call an expressman and forward 'em to that woman who was always tired!'

The Little Reporter looked up with a shrug of annoyance and protestation.

'Haven't ye got her address?' asked the boy, sympathetically, then quickly he added, 'Course not! She wouldn't give that, I guess, after all she told ye!'

They began to notice about the office that the Little Reporter in her corner was losing somewhat of her blithe look and manner. Her cheeks were paling and her eyes saddened and took on the look that comes of little sleep. In and out of the office, then intermittently at her desk, on which there now was scarce space for the moving of her pen, she worked on as was her custom, taking an assignment first here, then there, but her cheery laugh was now infrequent, and only occasionally came a flash of wit in her hurried conversations with the different members of the staff. They tried to joke her about the heroine of her story, but she failed to respond with her old-time lightning-like repartee.

'So those cuts have come at last!' exclaimed the assistant editor one afternoon as a messenger boy bore toward him an oblong cardboard box. He stretched out his hands for it. 'For "The Woman Who Was So Tired!" Please forward.' This was the inscription on the attached label, and on the box, in gold letters, 'Blank & Co., Florists – Broadway'.

'Hang "The Woman Who Was So Tired!"' he cried out angrily, then pointing to the desk where sat the Little Reporter, he added a bit softly, 'Take 'em over to that lady.'

She drew out from the box a dozen American Beauty roses, and hanging to the wide ribbon which bound their stems was a card. It read, 'From a tired man to a tired woman.'

She put them in the ice-water pitcher. They were beautiful roses and costly, and they shone out gloriously from among the heaps of parcels and letters addressed 'To the Woman Who Was So Tired'. The Little Reporter's fingers trembled on her pencil and a drop splashed down upon the yellow copy paper. For a moment her hand pressed her temple, then she dropped her face in her hands. The assistant editor walked over to her.

'Are you sick, Miss Sanderson?' he asked, kindly.

'No-o-o,' she drawled.

'I hope you haven't had some bad news?'

'No,' she said again. 'It's just about that "Woman Who Was So Tired". It's on my conscience. I can't rest – I – I –'

Nearly she broke down. Her eyes were growing big and shiny.

'All these letters, these bundles, these roses, oh! I didn't think it

7

would turn out like this – how could I know people would go on so? I had to get a story. I couldn't waste all that time – I hunted and searched until 9 o'clock that night, and I just—'

'Don't say you faked it,' interrupted the assistant editor. 'I know it's true; everybody knows it's true!'

'I didn't make it up. It was all true – oh, don't you understand? I was IT!'

Her face went down among the roses and the parcels.

The assistant editor gazed about the room, yet seeing none of the rush and the turmoil connected with getting out the next morning's paper, hearing none of the click of the typewriters nor the din at telegraph tables. And this was 'The Woman Who Was So Tired'! Their own Little Reporter, who went in and out among them, so unconsciously cheerful, so full of the joy of life and work, calling out sometimes when she had finished two columns, 'Find something else for me so I can run up a nice space bill this week!'

His mind travelled over the details of the story that had stirred so many hearts. The woman had appeared to be a book canvasser, working on commission – how like a reporter working on space and scouring the town for news! Frail and young, she had a whole family of dependents. In the story she had gone out in the ice and sleet, had slipped three times and turned her ankle. Instinctively he looked at the Little Reporter's feet and noticed that she was wearing odd shoes, the one shoe much larger than the other, doubtless because of the swelling of her sprained ankle. Why, on the night of the day when he had sent her out had she not returned laughing and limping?

He looked out of the window, out over the towering skyscrapers of great New York, where daily he had sent her to bring in news of the city's joys and sorrows, its weddings and its funerals, its prayers and its cursings, its virtue and its vice, its feasting and its fasting.

'The Woman Who Was So Tired' was often hungry! Had the Little Reporter ever lacked for food? Involuntarily his eye travelled back to her desk and rested upon the large-printed quotation one of the men reporters had jestingly hung above it the morning they had published her particularly racy and sparkling account of a banquet at Sherry's:

'Who writes the fine report of the feast? She who got none and enjoyed it least!'

For three years now the Little Reporter had been on his staff, the one woman among a dozen men. At first he had hesitated about taking her on, she had seemed so tiny, so young, so irresponsible. She had never spoken of her family, her home. Who would have suspected the burden she carried so lightly upon her slight shoulders? And on the day he had sent her out to write of the 'most anything woman' she could find in New York, surely there must have been some special reason at home why 'good space' was necessary to her that day! Once he had laughingly called her an Oliver Twist, because she was always 'asking for more' space. He had always suspected she spent large sums for clothes, for she dressed smartly with stylish gowns and nobby hats, but the woman of her story made her own dresses and hats on Sundays and after midnight! When did the Little Reporter get time to sleep?

From the high window he looked out again over busy, laughing, sorrowing, noisy, seething New York, then again at the head of the Little Reporter still sunk upon her desk, then around upon the men in the room.

'I expect,' he said to himself, 'we sometimes forget up here in our tower of observation that we, too, are a part of New York, and perhaps New York also forgets it. We're just a part, a part of it all, and how like we are, how very like!'

They were wanting him at his own desk and he hurried over, yet turning an instant to look again at the Little Reporter, and say a kindly word to reassure her troubled heart, he saw that her hand had fallen away from her face and that she was fast asleep in the midst of the hubbub of the Press room.

And he tripped off softly and motioned away Bobbie, who was hurrying to her with proofs, lest he disturb and awaken the woman who was so tired.

THE THREE GOLDEN APPLES

Nathaniel Hawthorne

D id you ever hear of the golden apples, that grew in the garden of the Hesperides? Ah, those were such apples as would bring a great price, by the bushel, if any of them could be found growing in the orchards of nowadays! But there is not, I suppose, a graft of that wonderful fruit on a single tree in the wide world. Not so much as a seed of those apples exists any longer.

And, even in the old, old, half-forgotten times, before the garden of the Hesperides was overrun with weeds, a great many people doubted whether there could be real trees that bore apples of solid gold upon their branches. All had heard of them, but nobody remembered to have seen any. Children, nevertheless, used to listen, open-mouthed, to stories of the golden apple-tree, and resolved to discover it, when they should be big enough. Adventurous young men, who desired to do a braver thing than any of their fellows, set out in quest of this fruit. Many of them returned no more; none of them brought back the apples. No wonder that they found it impossible to gather them! It is said that there was a dragon beneath the tree, with a hundred terrible heads, fifty of which were always on the watch, while the other fifty slept.

In my opinion it was hardly worth running so much risk for the sake of a solid golden apple. Had the apples been sweet, mellow and juicy, indeed that would be another matter. There might then have been some sense in trying to get at them, in spite of the hundred-headed dragon.

But, as I have already told you, it was quite a common thing with young persons, when tired of too much peace and rest, to go in search of the garden of the Hesperides. And once the adventure was undertaken by a hero who had enjoyed very little peace or rest since he came into the world. At the time of which I am going to speak, he was wandering through the pleasant land of Italy, with a mighty club in his hand, and a bow and quiver slung across his shoulders. He was wrapt in the skin of the biggest and fiercest lion that ever had been seen, and which he himself had killed; and though, on the whole, he was kind, and generous, and noble, there was a good deal of the lion's fierceness in his heart. As he went on his way, he continually inquired whether that were the right road to the famous garden. But none of the country people knew anything about the matter, and many looked as if they would have laughed at the question, if the stranger had not carried so very big a club.

So he journeyed on and on, still making the same inquiry, until, at last, he came to the brink of a river where some beautiful young women sat twining wreaths of flowers.

'Can you tell me, pretty maidens,' asked the stranger, 'whether this is the right way to the garden of the Hesperides?'

The young women had been having a fine time together, weaving the flowers into wreaths, and crowning one another's heads. And there seemed to be a kind of magic in the touch of their fingers, that made the flowers more fresh and dewy, and of brighter hues, and sweeter fragrance, while they played with them, than even when they had been growing on their native stems. But, on hearing the stranger's question, they dropped all their flowers on the grass, and gazed at him with astonishment.

'The garden of the Hesperides!' cried one. 'We thought mortals had been weary of seeking it, after so many disappointments. And pray, adventurous traveller, what do you want there?'

'A certain king, who is my cousin,' replied he, 'has ordered me to get him three of the golden apples.'

'Most of the young men who go in quest of these apples,' observed another of the damsels, 'desire to obtain them for themselves, or to present them to some fair maiden whom they love. Do you, then, love this king, your cousin, so very much?'

'Perhaps not,' replied the stranger, sighing. 'He has often been severe and cruel to me. But it is my destiny to obey him.'

'And do you know,' asked the damsel who had first spoken, 'that a terrible dragon, with a hundred heads, keeps watch under the golden apple-tree?'

'I know it well,' answered the stranger, calmly. 'But, from my cradle upwards, it has been my business, and almost my pastime, to deal with serpents and dragons.'

The young women looked at his massive club, and at the shaggy lion's skin which he wore, and likewise at his heroic limbs and figure; and they whispered to each other that the stranger appeared to be one who might reasonably expect to perform deeds far beyond the might of other men. But, then, the dragon with a hundred heads! What mortal, even if he possessed a hundred lives, could hope to escape the fangs of such a monster? So kind-hearted were the maidens, that they could not bear to see this brave and handsome traveller attempt what was so very dangerous, and devote himself, most probably, to become a meal for the dragon's hundred ravenous mouths.

'Go back,' cried they all – 'go back to your own home! Your mother, beholding you safe and sound, will shed tears of joy; and what can she do more, should you win ever so great a victory? No matter for the golden apples! No matter for the king, your cruel cousin! We do not wish the dragon with the hundred heads to eat you up!'

The stranger seemed to grow impatient at these remonstrances. He carelessly lifted his mighty club, and let it fall upon a rock that lay half buried in the earth, near by. With the force of that idle blow, the great rock was shattered all to pieces. It cost the stranger no more effort to achieve this feat of a giant's strength than for one of the young maidens to touch her sister's rosy cheek with a flower.

'Do you not believe,' said he, looking at the damsels with a smile, 'that such a blow would have crushed one of the dragon's hundred heads?'

Then he sat down on the grass, and told them the story of his life, or as much of it as he could remember, from the day when he was first cradled in a warrior's brazen shield. While he lay there, two immense serpents came gliding over the floor, and opened their hideous jaws to devour him; and he, a baby of a few months old, had gripped one of the fierce snakes in each of his little fists, and strangled them to death. When he was but a stripling, he had killed a huge lion, almost as big as the one whose vast and shaggy hide he now wore upon his shoulders. The next thing that he had done was to fight a battle with an ugly sort of monster, called a hydra, which had no less than nine heads, and exceedingly sharp teeth in every one.

'But the dragon of the Hesperides, you know,' observed one of the damsels, 'has a hundred heads!'

'Nevertheless,' replied the stranger, 'I would rather fight two such dragons than a single hydra. For, as fast as I cut off a head, two others grew in its place; and, besides, there was one of the heads that could not possibly be killed, but kept biting as fiercely as ever, long after it was cut off. So I was forced to bury it under a stone, where it is doubtless alive to this very day. But the hydra's body, and its eight other heads, will never do any further mischief.'

The damsels, judging that the story was likely to last a good while, had been preparing a repast of bread and grapes, that the stranger might refresh himself in the intervals of his talk. They took pleasure in helping him to this simple food; and, now and then, one of them would put a sweet grape between her rosy lips, lest it should make him bashful to eat alone.

The traveller proceeded to tell how he had chased a very swift stag, for a twelvemonth together, without ever stopping to take breath, and had at last caught it by the antlers, and carried it home alive. Besides all this, he took to himself great credit for having cleaned out a stable.

'Do you call that a wonderful exploit?' asked one of the young maidens, with a smile. 'Any clown in the country has done as much!'

'Had it been an ordinary stable,' replied the stranger, 'I should not have mentioned it. But this was so gigantic a task that it would have taken me all my life to perform it, if I had not luckily thought of turning the channel of a river through the stable-door. That did the business in a very short time!'

Seeing how earnestly his fair auditors listened, he next told them how he had shot some monstrous birds, and had caught a wild bull alive and let him go again, and had tamed a number of very wild horses, and had conquered Hippolyta, the warlike queen of the Amazons. He mentioned, likewise, that he had taken off Hippolyta's enchanted girdle, and had given it to the daughter of his cousin, the king.

'Was it the girdle of Venus,' inquired the prettiest of the damsels, 'which makes women beautiful?'

'No,' answered the stranger. 'It had formerly been the sword-belt of Mars; and it can only make the wearer valiant and courageous.'

'An old sword-belt!' cried the damsel, tossing her head. 'Then I should not care about having it!'

'You are right,' said the stranger.

Going on with his wonderful narrative, he informed the maidens that as strange an adventure as ever happened was when he fought with Geryon, the six-legged man. This was a very odd and frightful sort of figure, as you may well believe. Any person, looking at his tracks in the sand or snow, would suppose that three sociable companions had been walking along together. On hearing his footsteps at a little distance, it was no more than reasonable to judge that several people must be coming. But it was only the strange man Geryon clattering onward, with his six legs!

Six legs, and one gigantic body! Certainly, he must have been a very strange monster to look at; and, my stars, what a waste of shoe-leather!

When the stranger had finished the story of his adventures, he looked around at the attentive faces of the maidens.

'Perhaps you may have heard of me before,' said he, modestly. 'My name is Hercules!'

'We had already guessed it,' replied the maidens; 'for your wonderful deeds are known all over the world. We do not think it strange, any longer, that you should set out in quest of the golden apples of the Hesperides. Come, sisters, let us crown the hero with flowers!'

Then they flung beautiful wreaths over his stately head and mighty shoulders, so that the lion's skin was almost entirely covered with roses. They took possession of his ponderous club, and so entwined it about with the brightest, softest and most fragrant blossoms, that not a finger's breadth of its oaken substance could be seen. It looked all like a huge bunch of flowers. Lastly, they joined hands, and danced around him, chanting words which became poetry of their own accord, and grew into a choral song, in honour of the illustrious Hercules.

And Hercules was rejoiced, as any other hero would have been, to know that these fair young girls had heard of the valiant deeds which it had cost him so much toil and danger to achieve. But, still, he was not satisfied. He could not think that what he had already done was worthy of so much honour, while there remained any bold or difficult adventure to be undertaken.

'Dear maidens,' said he, when they paused to take breath, 'now that you know my name, will you not tell me how I am to reach the garden of the Hesperides?'

'Ah! must you go so soon?' they exclaimed. 'You – that have performed so many wonders, and spent such a toilsome life – cannot you content yourself to repose a little while on the margin of this peaceful river?'

Hercules shook his head.

'I must depart now,' said he.

'We will then give you the best directions we can,' replied the damsels. 'You must go to the sea-shore, and find out the Old One, and compel him to inform you where the golden apples are to be found.'

'The Old One!' repeated Hercules, laughing at this odd name. 'And, pray, who may the Old One be?'

'Why, the Old Man of the Sea, to be sure!' answered one of the damsels. 'He has fifty daughters, whom some people call very beautiful; but we do not think it proper to be acquainted with them, because they have sea-green hair, and taper away like fishes. You must talk with this Old Man of the Sea. He is a sea-faring person, and knows all about the garden of the Hesperides; for it is situated in an island which he is often in the habit of visiting.'

Hercules then asked whereabouts the Old One was most likely to be met with. When the damsels had informed him, he thanked them for all their kindness – for the bread and grapes with which they had fed him, the lovely flowers with which they had crowned him and the songs and dances wherewith they had done him honour – and he thanked them, most of all, for telling him the right way – and immediately set forth upon his journey.

But, before he was out of hearing, one of the maidens called after him.

'Keep fast hold of the Old One, when you catch him!' cried she, smiling, and lifting her finger to make the caution more impressive. 'Do not be astonished at anything that may happen. Only hold him fast, and he will tell you what you wish to know.'

Hercules again thanked her, and pursued his way, while the maidens resumed their pleasant labour of making flower-wreaths. They talked about the hero, long after he was gone.

'We will crown him with the loveliest of our garlands,' said they, 'when he returns hither with the three golden apples, after slaying the dragon with a hundred heads.'

Meanwhile, Hercules travelled constantly onward, over hill and dale, and through the solitary woods. Sometimes he swung his club aloft, and splintered a mighty oak with a downright blow. His mind was so full of the giants and monsters with whom it was the business of his life to fight, that perhaps he mistook the great tree for a giant or a monster. And so eager was Hercules to achieve what he had undertaken, that he almost regretted to have spent so much time with the damsels, wasting idle breath upon the story of his adventures. But thus it always is with persons who are destined to perform great things. What they have already done seems less than nothing. What they have taken in hand to do seems worth toil, danger and life itself.

Persons who happened to be passing through the forest must have been affrighted to see him smite the trees with his great club. With but a single blow, the trunk was riven as by the stroke of lightning, and the broad boughs came rustling and crashing down.

Hastening forward, without ever pausing or looking behind, he by and by heard the sea roaring at a distance. At this sound, he increased his speed, and soon came to a beach, where the great surf-waves tumbled themselves upon the hard sand, in a long line of snowy foam. At one end of the beach, however, there was a pleasant spot, where some green shrubbery clambered up a cliff, making its rocky face look soft and beautiful. A carpet of verdant grass, largely intermixed with sweet-smelling clover, covered the narrow space between the bottom of the cliff and the sea. And what should Hercules espy there, but an old man, fast asleep!

But was it really and truly an old man? Certainly, at first sight, it looked very like one; but, on closer inspection, it rather seemed to be some kind of a creature that lived in the sea. For, on his legs and arms there were scales, such as fishes have; he was web-footed and web-fingered, after the fashion of a duck; and his long beard, being of a greenish tinge, had more the appearance of a tuft of sea-weed than of an ordinary beard. Have you never seen a stick of timber, that has been long tossed about by the waves, and has got all overgrown with barnacles, and, at last drifting ashore, seems to have been thrown up from the very deepest bottom of the sea? Well, the old man would have put you in mind of just such a wave-tost spar! But Hercules, the instant he set eyes on this strange figure, was convinced that it could be no other than the Old One, who was to direct him on his way.

Yes, it was the selfsame Old Man of the Sea whom the hospitable maidens had talked to him about. Thanking his stars for the lucky accident of finding the old fellow asleep, Hercules stole on tiptoe towards him, and caught him by the arm and leg.

'Tell me,' cried he, before the Old One was well awake, 'which is the way to the garden of the Hesperides?'

As you may easily imagine, the Old Man of the Sea awoke in a fright. But his astonishment could hardly have been greater than was that of Hercules, the next moment. For, all of a sudden, the Old One seemed to disappear out of his grasp, and he found himself holding a stag by the fore and hind leg! But still he kept fast hold. Then the stag disappeared, and in its stead there was a sea-bird, fluttering and screaming, while Hercules clutched it by the wing and claw! But the bird could not get away. Immediately afterwards, there was an ugly three-headed dog, which growled and barked at Hercules, and snapped fiercely at the hands by which he held him! But Hercules would not let him go. In another minute, instead of the three-headed dog, what should appear but Geryon, the six-legged man-monster, kicking at Hercules with five of his legs, in order to get the remaining one at liberty! But Hercules held on. By and by, no Geryon was there, but a huge snake, like one of those which Hercules had strangled in his babyhood, only a hundred times as big; and it twisted and twined about the hero's neck and body, and threw its tail high into the air, and opened its deadly jaws as if to devour him outright; so that it was really a very terrible spectacle! But Hercules was no whit disheartened, and squeezed the great snake so tightly that he soon began to hiss with pain.

You must understand that the Old Man of the Sea, though he generally looked so much like the wave-beaten figure-head of a vessel, had the power of assuming any shape he pleased. When he found himself so roughly seized by Hercules, he had been in hopes of putting him into such surprise and terror, by these magical transformations, that the hero would be glad to let him go. If Hercules had relaxed his grasp, the Old One would certainly have plunged down to the very bottom of the sea, whence he would not soon have given himself the trouble of coming up, in order to answer any impertinent questions. Ninety-nine people out of a hundred, I suppose, would have been frightened out of their wits by the very first of his ugly shapes, and would have taken to their heels at once. For, one of the hardest things in this world is, to see the difference between real dangers and imaginary ones.

But, as Hercules held on so stubbornly, and only squeezed the Old One so much the tighter at every change of shape, and really put him to no small torture, he finally thought it best to reappear in his own figure. So there he was again, a fishy, scaly, web-footed sort of personage, with something like a tuft of sea-weed at his chin.

'Pray, what do you want with me?' cried the Old One, as soon as he could take breath; for it is quite a tiresome affair to go through so many false shapes. 'Why do you squeeze me so hard? Let me go, this moment, or I shall begin to consider you an extremely uncivil person!'

'My name is Hercules!' roared the mighty stranger. 'And you will never get out of my clutch, until you tell me the nearest way to the garden of the Hesperides!'

When the old fellow heard who it was that had caught him, he saw, with half an eye, that it would be necessary to tell him everything that he wanted to know. The Old One was an inhabitant of the sea, you must recollect, and roamed about everywhere, like other sea-faring people. Of course, he had often heard of the fame of Hercules, and of the wonderful things that he was constantly performing, in various parts of the earth, and how determined he always was to accomplish whatever he undertook. He therefore made no more attempts to escape, but told the hero how to find the garden of the Hesperides, and likewise warned him of many difficulties which must be overcome, before he could arrive thither.

'You must go on, thus and thus,' said the Old Man of the Sea, after taking the points of the compass, 'till you come in sight of a very tall giant, who holds the sky on his shoulders. And the giant, if he happens to be in the humour, will tell you exactly where the garden of the Hesperides lies.'

'And if the giant happens not to be in the humour,' remarked Hercules, balancing his club on the tip of his finger, 'perhaps I shall find means to persuade him!'

Thanking the Old Man of the Sea, and begging his pardon for having squeezed him so roughly, the hero resumed his journey. He met with a great many strange adventures, which would be well worth your hearing, if I had leisure to narrate them as minutely as they deserve.

It was in this journey, if I mistake not, that he encountered a prodigious giant, who was so wonderfully contrived by nature, that, every time he touched the earth, he became ten times as strong as ever he had been before. His name was Antæus. You may see, plainly enough, that it was a very difficult business to fight with such a fellow; for, as often as he got a knock-down blow, up he started again, stronger, fiercer and abler to use his weapons, than if his enemy had let him alone. Thus, the harder Hercules pounded the giant with his club, the further he seemed from winning the victory. I have sometimes argued with such people, but never fought with one. The only way in which Hercules found it possible to finish the battle, was by lifting Antæus off his feet into the air, and squeezing, and squeezing, and squeezing him, until, finally, the strength was quite squeezed out of his enormous body.

When this affair was finished, Hercules continued his travels, and went to the land of Egypt, where he was taken prisoner, and would have been put to death, if he had not slain the king of the country, and made his escape. Passing through the deserts of Africa, and going as fast as he could, he arrived at last on the shore of the great ocean. And here, unless he could walk on the crests of the billows, it seemed as if his journey must needs be at an end.

Nothing was before him, save the foaming, dashing, measureless ocean. But, suddenly, as he looked towards the horizon, he saw something, a great way off, which he had not seen the moment before. It gleamed very brightly, almost as you may have beheld the round, golden disk of the sun, when it rises or sets over the edge of the world. It evidently drew nearer; for, at every instant, this wonderful object became larger and more lustrous. At length, it had come so nigh that Hercules discovered it to be an immense cup or bowl, made either of gold or burnished brass. How it had got afloat upon the sea is more than I can tell you. There it was, at all events, rolling on the tumultuous billows, which tossed it up and down, and heaved their foamy tops against its sides, but without ever throwing their spray over the brim.

'I have seen many giants, in my time,' thought Hercules, 'but never one that would need to drink his wine out of a cup like this!'

And, true enough, what a cup it must have been! It was as large – as large – but, in short, I am afraid to say how immeasurably large it was. To speak within bounds, it was ten times larger than a great mill-wheel; and, all of metal as it was, it floated over the heaving surges more lightly than an acorn-cup adown the brook. The waves tumbled it onward, until it grazed against the shore, within a short distance of the spot where Hercules was standing.

As soon as this happened, he knew what was to be done; for he had not gone through so many remarkable adventures without learning pretty well how to conduct himself, whenever anything came to pass a little out of the common rule. It was just as clear as daylight that this marvellous cup had been set adrift by some unseen power, and guided hitherward, in order to carry Hercules across the sea, on his way to the garden of the Hesperides. Accordingly, without a moment's delay, he clambered over the brim, and slid down on the inside, where, spreading out his lion's skin, he proceeded to take a little repose. He had scarcely rested, until now, since he bade farewell to the damsels on the margin of the river. The waves dashed, with a pleasant and ringing sound, against the circumference of the hollow cup; it rocked lightly to and fro, and the motion was so soothing that it speedily rocked Hercules into an agreeable slumber.

His nap had probably lasted a good while, when the cup chanced to graze against a rock, and, in consequence, immediately resounded and reverberated through its golden or brazen substance, a hundred times as loudly as ever you heard a church-bell. The noise awoke Hercules, who instantly started up and gazed around him, wondering whereabouts he was. He was not long in discovering that the cup had floated across a great part of the sea, and was approaching the shore of what seemed to be an island. And, on that island, what do you think he saw?

No; you will never guess it, not if you were to try fifty thousand times! It positively appears to me that this was the most marvellous spectacle that had ever been seen by Hercules, in the whole course of his wonderful travels and adventures. It was a greater marvel than the hydra with nine heads, which kept growing twice as fast as they were cut off; greater than the six-legged man-monster; greater than Antæus; greater than anything that was ever beheld by anybody, before or since the days of Hercules, or than anything that remains to be beheld, by travellers in all time to come. It was a giant!

But such an intolerably big giant! A giant as tall as a mountain; so vast a giant, that the clouds rested about his midst, like a girdle, and hung like a hoary beard from his chin, and flitted before his huge eyes, so that he could neither see Hercules nor the golden cup in which he was voyaging. And, most wonderful of all, the giant held up his great hands and appeared to support the sky, which, so far as Hercules could discern through the clouds, was resting upon his head! This does really seem almost too much to believe.

Meanwhile, the bright cup continued to float onward, and finally touched the strand. Just then a breeze wafted away the clouds from before the giant's visage, and Hercules beheld it, with all its enormous features; eyes each of them as big as yonder lake, a nose a mile long and a mouth of the same width. It was a countenance terrible from its enormity of size, but disconsolate and weary, even as you may see the faces of many people, nowadays, who are compelled to sustain burdens above their strength. What the sky was to the giant, such are the cares of earth to those who let themselves be weighed down by them. And whenever men undertake what is beyond the just measure of their abilities, they encounter precisely such a doom as had befallen this poor giant.

Poor fellow! He had evidently stood there a long while. An ancient forest had been growing and decaying around his feet; and oak-trees, of six or seven centuries old, had sprung from the acorn, and forced themselves between his toes.

The giant now looked down from the far height of his great eyes, and, perceiving Hercules, roared out, in a voice that resembled thunder, proceeding out of the cloud that had just flitted away from his face.

'Who are you, down at my feet there? And whence do you come, in that little cup?'

'I am Hercules!' thundered back the hero, in a voice pretty nearly or quite as loud as the giant's own. 'And I am seeking for the garden of the Hesperides!'

'Ho! ho! ho!' roared the giant, in a fit of immense laughter. 'That is a wise adventure, truly!'

'And why not?' cried Hercules, getting a little angry at the giant's mirth. 'Do you think I am afraid of the dragon with a hundred heads!'

Just at this time, while they were talking together, some black clouds gathered about the giant's middle, and burst into a tremendous storm of thunder and lightning, causing such a pother that Hercules found it impossible to distinguish a word. Only the giant's immeasurable legs were to be seen, standing up into the obscurity of the tempest; and, now and then, a momentary glimpse of his whole figure, mantled in a volume of mist. He seemed to be speaking, most of the time; but his big, deep, rough voice chimed in with the reverberations of the thunder-claps, and rolled away over the hills, like them. Thus, by talking out of season, the foolish giant expended an incalculable quantity of breath, to no purpose; for the thunder spoke quite as intelligibly as he.

At last, the storm swept over, as suddenly as it had come. And there again was the clear sky, and the weary giant holding it up, and the pleasant sunshine beaming over his vast height, and illuminating it against the background of the sullen thunderclouds. So far above the shower had been his head, that not a hair of it was moistened by the rain-drops!

When the giant could see Hercules still standing on the sea-shore, he roared out to him anew.

'I am Atlas, the mightiest giant in the world! And I hold the sky upon my head!'

'So I see,' answered Hercules. 'But, can you show me the way to the garden of the Hesperides?'

'What do you want there?' asked the giant.

'I want three of the golden apples,' shouted Hercules, 'for my cousin, the king.'

'There is nobody but myself,' quoth the giant, 'that can go to the garden of the Hesperides, and gather the golden apples. If it were not for this little business of holding up the sky, I would make half a dozen steps across the sea, and get them for you.'

'You are very kind,' replied Hercules. 'And cannot you rest the sky upon a mountain?'

'None of them are quite high enough,' said Atlas, shaking his head. 'But, if you were to take your stand on the summit of that nearest one, your head would be pretty nearly on a level with mine. You seem to be a fellow of some strength. What if you should take my burden on your shoulders, while I do your errand for you?'

Hercules, as you must be careful to remember, was a remarkably strong man; and though it certainly requires a great deal of muscular power to uphold the sky, yet, if any mortal could be supposed capable of such an exploit, he was the one. Nevertheless, it seemed so difficult an undertaking, that, for the first time in his life, he hesitated.

'Is the sky very heavy?' he inquired.

'Why, not particularly so, at first,' answered the giant, shrugging his shoulders. 'But it gets to be a little burdensome, after a thousand years!'

'And how long a time,' asked the hero, 'will it take you to get the golden apples?'

'Oh, that will be done in a few moments,' cried Atlas. 'I shall take ten or fifteen miles at a stride, and be at the garden and back again before your shoulders begin to ache.'

'Well, then,' answered Hercules, 'I will climb the mountain behind you there, and relieve you of your burden.'

The truth is, Hercules had a kind heart of his own, and considered that he should be doing the giant a favour, by allowing him this opportunity for a ramble. And, besides, he thought that it would be still more for his own glory, if he could boast of upholding the sky, than merely to do so ordinary a thing as to conquer a dragon with a hundred heads. Accordingly, without more words, the sky was shifted from the shoulders of Atlas, and placed upon those of Hercules.

When this was safely accomplished, the first thing that the giant did was to stretch himself; and you may imagine what a prodigious spectacle he was then. Next, he slowly lifted one of his feet out of the forest that had grown up around it; then, the other. Then, all at once, he began to caper, and leap, and dance, for joy at his freedom; flinging himself nobody knows how high into the air, and floundering down again with a shock that made the earth tremble. Then he laughed – Ho! ho! ho! – with a thunderous roar that was echoed from the mountains, far and near, as if they and the giant had been so many rejoicing brothers. When his joy had a little subsided, he stepped into the sea; ten miles at the first stride, which brought him midleg deep; and ten miles at the second, when the water came just above his knees; and ten miles more at the third, by which he was immersed nearly to his waist. This was the greatest depth of the sea.

Hercules watched the giant, as he still went onward; for it was really a wonderful sight, this immense human form, more than thirty miles off, half hidden in the ocean, but with his upper half as tall, and misty, and blue, as a distant mountain. At last the gigantic shape faded entirely out of view. And now Hercules began to consider what he should do, in case Atlas should be drowned in the sea, or if he were to be stung to death by the dragon with the hundred heads, which guarded the golden apples of the Hesperides. If any such misfortune were to happen, how could he ever get rid of the sky? And, by the by, its weight began already to be a little irksome to his head and shoulders.

'I really pity the poor giant,' thought Hercules. 'If it wearies me so much in ten minutes, how must it have wearied him in a thousand years!'

O my sweet little people, you have no idea what a weight there was in that same blue sky, which looks so soft and aerial above our heads! And there, too, was the bluster of the wind, and the chill and watery clouds, and the blazing sun, all taking their turns to make Hercules uncomfortable! He began to be afraid that the giant would never come back. He gazed wistfully at the world beneath him, and acknowledged to himself that it was a far happier kind of life to be a shepherd at the foot of a mountain, than to stand on its dizzy summit, and bear up the firmament with his might and main. For, of course, as you will easily understand, Hercules had an immense responsibility on his mind, as well as a weight on his head and shoulders. Why, if he did not stand perfectly still, and keep the sky immovable, the sun would perhaps be put ajar! Or, after nightfall, a great many of the stars might be loosened from their places, and shower down, like fiery rain, upon the people's heads! And how ashamed would the hero be, if, owing to his unsteadiness beneath its weight, the sky should crack, and show a great fissure quite across it!

I know not how long it was before, to his unspeakable joy, he beheld the huge shape of the giant, like a cloud, on the far-off edge of the sea. At his nearer approach, Atlas held up his hand, in which Hercules could perceive three magnificent golden apples, as big as pumpkins, all hanging from one branch.

'I am glad to see you again,' shouted Hercules, when the giant was within hearing. 'So you have got the golden apples?'

'Certainly, certainly,' answered Atlas; 'and very fair apples they are. I took the finest that grew on the tree, I assure you. Ah! it is a beautiful spot, that garden of the Hesperides. Yes; and the dragon with a hundred heads is a sight worth any man's seeing. After all, you had better have gone for the apples yourself.'

'No matter,' replied Hercules. 'You have had a pleasant ramble, and have done the business as well as I could. I heartily thank you for your trouble. And now, as I have a long way to go, and am rather in haste – and as the king, my cousin, is anxious to receive the golden apples – will you be kind enough to take the sky off my shoulders again?'

'Why, as to that,' said the giant, chucking the golden apples into the air twenty miles high, or thereabouts, and catching them as they came down – 'as to that, my good friend, I consider you a little unreasonable. Cannot I carry the golden apples to the king, your cousin, much quicker than you could? As his majesty is in such a hurry to get them, I promise you to take my longest strides. And, besides, I have no fancy for burdening myself with the sky, just now.'

Here Hercules grew impatient, and gave a great shrug of his shoulders. It being now twilight, you might have seen two or three stars tumble out of their places. Everybody on earth looked upward in affright, thinking that the sky might be going to fall next.

'Oh, that will never do!' cried Giant Atlas, with a great roar of laughter. 'I have not let fall so many stars within the last five centuries. By the time you have stood there as long as I did, you will begin to learn patience!'

'What!' shouted Hercules, very wrathfully, 'do you intend to make me bear this burden forever?'

'We will see about that, one of these days,' answered the giant. 'At all events, you ought not to complain, if you have to bear it the next hundred years, or perhaps the next thousand. I bore it a good while longer, in spite of the back-ache. Well, then, after a thousand years, if I happen to feel in the mood, we may possibly shift about again. You are certainly a very strong man, and can never have a better opportunity to prove it. Posterity will talk of you, I warrant it!'

'Pish! a fig for its talk!' cried Hercules, with another hitch of his shoulders. 'Just take the sky upon your head one instant, will you? I want to make a cushion of my lion's skin, for the weight to rest upon. It really chafes me, and will cause unnecessary inconvenience in so many centuries as I am to stand here.'

'That's no more than fair, and I'll do it!' quoth the giant; for he had no unkind feeling towards Hercules, and was merely acting with a too selfish consideration of his own ease. 'For just five minutes, then, I'll take back the sky. Only for five minutes, recollect! I have no idea of spending another thousand years as I spent the last. Variety is the spice of life, say I.'

Ah, the thick-witted old rogue of a giant! He threw down the golden apples, and received back the sky, from the head and shoulders of Hercules, upon his own, where it rightly belonged. And Hercules picked up the three golden apples, that were as big or bigger than pumpkins, and straightway set out on his journey homeward, without paying the slightest heed to the thundering tones of the giant, who bellowed after him to come back. Another forest sprang up around his feet, and grew ancient there; and again might be seen oak-trees, of six or seven centuries old, that had waxed thus aged betwixt his enormous toes.

And there stands the giant to this day; or, at any rate, there stands a mountain as tall as he, and which bears his name; and when the thunder rumbles about its summit, we may imagine it to be the voice of Giant Atlas, bellowing after Hercules!

HER FIRST BALL

Katherine Mansfield

Exactly when the ball began Leila would have found it hard to say. Perhaps her first real partner was the cab. It did not matter that she shared the cab with the Sheridan girls and their brother. She sat back in her own little corner of it, and the bolster on which her hand rested felt like the sleeve of an unknown young man's dress suit; and away they bowled, past waltzing lamp-posts and houses and fences and trees.

'Have you really never been to a ball before, Leila? But, my child, how too weird—' cried the Sheridan girls.

'Our nearest neighbour was fifteen miles,' said Leila softly, gently opening and shutting her fan.

Oh dear, how hard it was to be indifferent like the others! She tried not to smile too much; she tried not to care. But every single thing was so new and exciting . . . Meg's tuberoses, Jose's long loop of amber, Laura's little dark head, pushing above her white fur like a flower through snow. She would remember for ever. It even gave her a pang to see her cousin Laurie throw away the wisps of tissue paper he pulled from the fastenings of his new gloves. She would like to have kept those wisps as a keepsake, as a remembrance. Laurie leaned forward and put his hand on Laura's knee.

'Look here, darling,' he said. 'The third and the ninth as usual. Twig?'

Oh, how marvellous to have a brother! In her excitement Leila felt that if there had been time, if it hadn't been impossible, she couldn't have helped crying because she was an only child, and no brother had ever said 'Twig?' to her; no sister would ever say, as Meg said to Jose that moment, 'I've never known your hair go up more successfully than it has to-night!'

But, of course, there was no time. They were at the drill hall already; there were cabs in front of them and cabs behind. The road was bright on either side with moving fan-like lights, and on the pavement gay couples seemed to float through the air; little satin shoes chased each other like birds.

'Hold on to me, Leila; you'll get lost,' said Laura.

'Come on, girls, let's make a dash for it,' said Laurie.

Leila put two fingers on Laura's pink velvet cloak, and they were somehow lifted past the big golden lantern, carried along the passage and pushed into the little room marked 'Ladies'. Here the crowd was so great there was hardly space to take off their things; the noise was deafening. Two benches on either side were stacked high with wraps. Two old women in white aprons ran up and down tossing fresh armfuls. And everybody was pressing forward trying to get at the little dressing-table and mirror at the far end.

A great quivering jet of gas lighted the ladies' room. It couldn't wait; it was dancing already. When the door opened again and there came a burst of tuning from the drill hall, it leaped almost to the ceiling.

Dark girls, fair girls were patting their hair, tying ribbons again, tucking handkerchiefs down the fronts of their bodices, smoothing marble-white gloves. And because they were all laughing it seemed to Leila that they were all lovely.

'Aren't there any invisible hair-pins?' cried a voice. 'How most extraordinary! I can't see a single invisible hair-pin.'

'Powder my back, there's a darling,' cried some one else.

'But I must have a needle and cotton. I've torn simply miles and miles of the frill,' wailed a third.

Then, 'Pass them along, pass them along!' The straw basket of programmes was tossed from arm to arm. Darling little pink-and-silver programmes, with pink pencils and fluffy tassels. Leila's fingers shook as she took one out of the basket. She wanted to ask some one, 'Am I meant to have one too?' but she had just time to read: 'Waltz 3. "Two, Two in a Canoe." Polka 4. "Making the Feathers Fly,"' when Meg cried, 'Ready, Leila?' and they pressed their way through the crush in the passage towards the big double doors of the drill hall.

Dancing had not begun yet, but the band had stopped tuning, and the noise was so great it seemed that when it did begin to play it would never be heard. Leila, pressing close to Meg, looking over Meg's shoulder, felt that even the little quivering coloured flags strung across the ceiling were talking. She quite forgot to be shy; she forgot how in the middle of dressing she had sat down on the bed with one shoe off and one shoe on and begged her mother to ring up her cousins and say she couldn't go after all. And the rush of longing she had had to be sitting on the veranda of their forsaken up-country home, listening to the baby owls crying 'More pork' in the moonlight, was changed to a rush of joy so sweet that it was hard to bear alone. She clutched her fan, and, gazing at the gleaming, golden floor, the azaleas, the lanterns, the stage at one end with its red carpet and gilt chairs and the band in a corner, she thought breathlessly, 'How heavenly; how simply heavenly!'

All the girls stood grouped together at one side of the doors, the men at the other, and the chaperones in dark dresses, smiling rather foolishly, walked with little careful steps over the polished floor towards the stage.

'This is my little country cousin Leila. Be nice to her. Find her partners; she's under my wing,' said Meg, going up to one girl after another.

Strange faces smiled at Leila – sweetly, vaguely. Strange voices answered, 'Of course, my dear.' But Leila felt the girls didn't really see her. They were looking towards the men. Why didn't the men begin? What were they waiting for? There they stood, smoothing their gloves, patting their glossy hair and smiling among themselves. Then, quite suddenly, as if they had only just made up their minds that that was what they had to do, the men came gliding over the parquet. There was a joyful flutter among the girls. A tall, fair man flew up to Meg, seized her programme, scribbled something; Meg passed him on to Leila. 'May I have the pleasure?' He ducked and smiled. There came a dark man wearing an eyeglass, then cousin Laurie with a friend, and Laura with a little freckled fellow whose tie was crooked. Then quite an old man – fat, with a big bald patch on his head – took her programme and murmured, 'Let me see, let me see!' And he was a long time comparing his programme, which looked black with names, with hers. It seemed to give him so much trouble that Leila was ashamed. 'Oh, please don't bother,' she said eagerly. But instead of replying the fat man wrote something, glanced at her again. 'Do I remember this bright little face?' he said softly. 'Is it known to me of yore?' At that moment the band began playing; the fat man disappeared. He was tossed away on a great wave of music that came flying over the gleaming floor, breaking the groups up into couples, scattering them, sending them spinning . . .

Leila had learned to dance at boarding school. Every Saturday afternoon the boarders were hurried off to a little corrugated iron mission hall where Miss Eccles (of London) held her 'select' classes. But the difference between that dusty-smelling hall – with calico texts on the walls, the poor terrified little woman in a brown velvet toque with rabbit's ears thumping the cold piano, Miss Eccles poking the girls' feet with her long white wand – and this was so tremendous that Leila was sure if her partner didn't come and she had to listen to that marvellous music and to watch the others sliding, gliding over the golden floor, she would die at least, or faint, or lift her arms and fly out of one of those dark windows that showed the stars.

'Ours, I think—' Some one bowed, smiled and offered her his arm; she hadn't to die after all. Some one's hand pressed her waist, and she floated away like a flower that is tossed into a pool.

'Quite a good floor, isn't it?' drawled a faint voice close to her ear.

'I think it's most beautifully slippery,' said Leila.

'Pardon!' The faint voice sounded surprised. Leila said it again. And there was a tiny pause before the voice echoed, 'Oh, quite!' and she was swung round again.

He steered so beautifully. That was the great difference between dancing with girls and men, Leila decided. Girls banged into each other, and stamped on each other's feet; the girl who was gentleman always clutched you so.

The azaleas were separate flowers no longer; they were pink and white flags streaming by.

'Were you at the Bells' last week?' the voice came again. It sounded tired. Leila wondered whether she ought to ask him if he would like to stop.

'No, this is my first dance,' said she.

Her partner gave a little gasping laugh. 'Oh, I say,' he protested.

'Yes, it is really the first dance I've ever been to.' Leila was most fervent. It was such a relief to be able to tell somebody. 'You see, I've lived in the country all my life up till now . . .'

At that moment the music stopped, and they went to sit on two chairs against the wall. Leila tucked her pink satin feet under and fanned herself, while she blissfully watched the other couples passing and disappearing through the swing doors.

'Enjoying yourself, Leila?' asked Jose, nodding her golden head.

Laura passed and gave her the faintest little wink; it made Leila wonder for a moment whether she was quite grown up after all. Certainly her partner did not say very much. He coughed, tucked his handkerchief away, pulled down his waistcoat, took a minute thread off his sleeve. But it didn't matter. Almost immediately the band started and her second partner seemed to spring from the ceiling.

'Floor's not bad,' said the new voice. Did one always begin with the floor? And then, 'Were you at the Neaves' on Tuesday?' And again Leila explained. Perhaps it was a little strange that her partners were not more interested. For it was thrilling. Her first ball! She was only at the beginning of everything. It seemed to her that she had never known what the night was like before. Up till now it had been dark, silent, beautiful very often – oh yes – but mournful somehow. Solemn. And now it would never be like that again – it had opened dazzling bright.

'Care for an ice?' said her partner. And they went through the swing doors, down the passage, to the supper room. Her cheeks burned, she was fearfully thirsty. How sweet the ices looked on little glass plates and how cold the frosted spoon was, iced too! And when they came back to the hall there was the fat man waiting for her by the door. It gave her quite a shock again to see how old he was; he ought to have been on the stage with the fathers and mothers. And when Leila compared him with her other partners he looked shabby. His waistcoat was creased, there was a button off his glove, his coat looked as if it was dusty with French chalk.

'Come along, little lady,' said the fat man. He scarcely troubled to clasp her, and they moved away so gently, it was more like walking than dancing. But he said not a word about the floor. 'Your first dance, isn't it?' he murmured.

'How did you know?'

'Ah,' said the fat man, 'that's what it is to be old!' He wheezed faintly as he steered her past an awkward couple. 'You see, I've been doing this kind of thing for the last thirty years.'

'Thirty years?' cried Leila. Twelve years before she was born!

'It hardly bears thinking about, does it?' said the fat man gloomily. Leila looked at his bald head, and she felt quite sorry for him.

'I think it's marvellous to be still going on,' she said kindly.

'Kind little lady,' said the fat man, and he pressed her a little closer, and hummed a bar of the waltz. 'Of course,' he said, 'you can't hope to last anything like as long as that. No-o,' said the fat man, 'long before that you'll be sitting up there on the stage, looking on, in your nice black velvet. And these pretty arms will have turned into little short fat ones, and you'll beat time with such a different kind of fan – a black bony one.' The fat man seemed to shudder. 'And you'll smile away like the poor old dears up there, and point to your daughter, and tell the elderly lady next to you how some dreadful man tried to kiss her at the club ball. And your heart will ache, ache' – the fat man squeezed her closer still, as if he really was sorry for that poor heart – 'because no one wants to kiss you now. And you'll say how unpleasant these polished floors are to walk on, how dangerous they are. Eh, Mademoiselle Twinkletoes?' said the fat man softly.

Leila gave a light little laugh, but she did not feel like laughing. Was it – could it all be true? It sounded terribly true. Was this first ball only the beginning of her last ball, after all? At that the music seemed to change; it sounded sad, sad; it rose upon a great sigh. Oh, how quickly things changed! Why didn't happiness last for ever? For ever wasn't a bit too long.

'I want to stop,' she said in a breathless voice. The fat man led her to the door.

'No,' she said, 'I won't go outside. I won't sit down. I'll just stand here, thank you.' She leaned against the wall, tapping with her foot, pulling up her gloves and trying to smile. But deep inside her a little girl threw her pinafore over her head and sobbed. Why had he spoiled it all?

'I say, you know,' said the fat man, 'you mustn't take me seriously, little lady.'

'As if I should!' said Leila, tossing her small dark head and sucking her underlip . . .

Again the couples paraded. The swing doors opened and shut. Now new music was given out by the bandmaster. But Leila didn't want to dance any more. She wanted to be home, or sitting on the veranda listening to those baby owls. When she looked through the dark windows at the stars, they had long beams like wings . . .

But presently a soft, melting, ravishing tune began, and a young man with curly hair bowed before her. She would have to dance, out of politeness, until she could find Meg. Very stiffly she walked into the middle; very haughtily she put her hand on his sleeve. But in one minute, in one turn, her feet glided, glided. The lights, the azaleas, the dresses, the pink faces, the velvet chairs, all became one beautiful flying wheel. And when her next partner bumped her into the fat man and he said, 'Pardon,' she smiled at him more radiantly than ever. She didn't even recognize him again.

LOVE IN THE NIGHT

F Scott Fitzgerald

I

The words thrilled Val. They had come into his mind sometime during the fresh gold April afternoon and he kept repeating them to himself over and over: 'Love in the night; love in the night.' He tried them in three languages – Russian, French and English – and decided that they were best in English. In each language they meant a different sort of love and a different sort of night – the English night seemed the warmest and softest with a thinnest and most crystalline sprinkling of stars. The English love seemed the most fragile and romantic – a white dress and a dim face above it and eyes that were pools of light. And when I add that it was a French night he was thinking about, after all, I see I must go back and begin over.

Val was half Russian and half American. His mother was the daughter of that Morris Hasylton who helped finance the Chicago World's Fair in 1892, and his father was – see the Almanach de Gotha, issue of 1910 – Prince Paul Serge Boris Rostoff, son of Prince Vladimir Rostoff, grandson of a grand duke – 'Jimber-jawed Serge' – and third-cousin-once-removed to the czar. It was all very impressive, you see, on that side – house in St Petersburg, shooting lodge near Riga and swollen villa, more like a palace, overlooking the Mediterranean. It was at this villa in Cannes that the Rostoffs passed the winter – and it wasn't at all the thing to remind Princess Rostoff that this Riviera villa, from the marble fountain – after Bernini – to the gold cordial glasses – after dinner – was paid for with American gold.

The Russians, of course, were lively people on the Continent in the gala days before the war. Of the three races that used Southern France for a pleasure ground they were easily the most adept at the grand manner. The English were too practical, and the Americans, though they spent freely, had no tradition of romantic conduct. But the Russians – there was a people as gallant as the Latins, and rich besides! When the Rostoffs arrived at Cannes late in January the restaurateurs telegraphed north for the Prince's favourite labels to paste on their champagne, and the jewellers put incredibly gorgeous articles aside to show to him – but not to the princess – and the Russian Church was swept and garnished for the season that the Prince might beg orthodox forgiveness for his sins. Even the Mediterranean turned obligingly to a deep wine colour in the spring evenings, and fishing boats with robin-breasted sails loitered exquisitely offshore.

In a vague way young Val realized that this was all for the benefit of him and his family. It was a privileged paradise, this white little city on the water, in which he was free to do what he liked because he was rich and young and the blood of Peter the Great ran indigo in his veins. He was only seventeen in 1914, when this history begins, but he had already fought a duel with a young man four years his senior, and he had a small hairless scar to show for it on top of his handsome head.

But the question of love in the night was the thing nearest his heart. It was a vague pleasant dream he had, something that was going to happen to him some day that would be unique and incomparable. He could have told no more about it than that there was a lovely unknown girl concerned in it, and that it ought to take place beneath the Riviera moon.

The odd thing about all this was not that he had this excited and yet almost spiritual hope of romance, for all boys of any imagination have just such hopes, but that it actually came true. And when it happened, it happened so unexpectedly; it was such a jumble of impressions and emotions, of curious phrases that sprang to his lips, of sights and sounds and moments that were here, were lost, were past, that he scarcely understood it at all. Perhaps its very vagueness preserved it in his heart and made him forever unable to forget.

There was an atmosphere of love all about him that spring – his father's loves, for instance, which were many and indiscreet, and which Val became aware of gradually from overhearing the gossip of servants, and definitely from coming on his American mother unexpectedly one afternoon, to find her storming hysterically at his father's picture on the salon wall. In the picture his father wore a white uniform with a furred dolman and looked back impassively at his wife as if to say 'Were you under the impression, my dear, that you were marrying into a family of clergymen?'

Val tiptoed away, surprised, confused – and excited. It didn't shock him as it would have shocked an American boy of his age. He had known for years what life was among the Continental rich, and he condemned his father only for making his mother cry.

Love went on around him – reproachless love and illicit love alike. As he strolled along the seaside promenade at nine o'clock, when the stars were bright enough to compete with the bright lamps, he was aware of love on every side. From the open-air cafés, vivid with dresses just down from Paris, came a sweet pungent odour of flowers and chartreuse and fresh black coffee and cigarettes – and mingled with them all he caught another scent, the mysterious thrilling scent of love. Hands touched jewel-sparkling hands upon the white tables. Bright dresses and white shirt fronts swayed together, and matches were held, trembling a little, for slow-lighting cigarettes. On the other side of the boulevard lovers less fashionable, young Frenchmen who worked in the stores of Cannes, sauntered with their fiancées under the dim trees, but Val's young eyes seldom turned that way. The luxury of music and bright colours and low voices – they were all part of his dream. They were the essential trappings of love in the night.

But assume as he might the rather fierce expression that was expected from a young Russian gentleman who walked the streets alone, Val was beginning to be unhappy. April twilight had succeeded March twilight, the season was almost over, and he had found no use to make of the warm spring evenings. The girls of sixteen and seventeen whom he knew, were chaperoned with care between dusk and bedtime – this, remember, was before the war – and the others who might gladly have walked beside him were an affront to his romantic desire. So April passed by – one week, two weeks, three weeks—

He had played tennis until seven and loitered at the courts for another hour, so it was half-past eight when a tired cab horse accomplished the hill on which gleamed the façade of the Rostoff villa. The lights of his mother's limousine were yellow in the drive, and the princess, buttoning her gloves, was just coming out the glowing door. Val tossed two francs to the cabman and went to kiss her on the cheek.

'Don't touch me,' she said quickly. 'You've been handling money.'

'But not in my mouth, mother,' he protested humorously.

The princess looked at him impatiently.

'I'm angry,' she said. 'Why must you be so late tonight? We're dining on a yacht and you were to have come along too.'

'What yacht?'

'Americans.' There was always a faint irony in her voice when she mentioned the land of her nativity. Her America was the Chicago of the nineties which she still thought of as the vast upstairs to a butcher shop. Even the irregularities of Prince Paul were not too high a price to have paid for her escape.

'Two yachts,' she continued; 'in fact we don't know which one. The note was very indefinite. Very careless indeed.'

Americans. Val's mother had taught him to look down on Americans, but she hadn't succeeded in making him dislike them. American men noticed you, even if you were seventeen. He liked Americans. Although he was thoroughly Russian he wasn't immaculately so – the exact proportion, like that of a celebrated soap, was about ninety-nine and three-quarters per cent.

'I want to come,' he said, 'I'll hurry up, mother. I'll—'

'We're late now.' The princess turned as her husband appeared in the door. 'Now Val says he wants to come.'

'He can't,' said Prince Paul shortly. 'He's too outrageously late.'

Val nodded. Russian aristocrats, however indulgent about themselves, were always admirably Spartan with their children. There were no arguments.

'I'm sorry,' he said.

Prince Paul grunted. The footman, in red and silver livery, opened the limousine door. But the grunt decided the matter for Val, because Princess Rostoff at that day and hour had certain grievances against her husband which gave her command of the domestic situation.

'On second thought you'd better come, Val,' she announced coolly. 'It's too late now, but come after dinner. The yacht is either the Minnehaha or the Privateer.' She got into the limousine. 'The one to come to will be the jolly one, I suppose – the Jacksons' yacht—'

'Find got sense,' muttered the Prince cryptically, conveying that

Val would find it if he had any sense. 'Have my man take a look at you 'fore you start. Wear tie of mine 'stead of that outrageous string you affected in Vienna. Grow up. High time.'

As the limousine crawled crackling down the pebbled drive Val's face was burning.

II

It was dark in Cannes harbour; rather it seemed dark after the brightness of the promenade that Val had just left behind. Three frail dock lights glittered dimly upon innumerable fishing boats heaped like shells along the beach. Farther out in the water there were other lights where a fleet of slender yachts rode the tide with slow dignity, and farther still a full ripe moon made the water bosom into a polished dancing floor. Occasionally there was a swish! creak! drip! as a rowboat moved about in the shallows, and its blurred shape threaded the labyrinth of hobbled fishing skiffs and launches. Val, descending the velvet slope of sand, stumbled over a sleeping boatman and caught the rank savour of garlic and plain wine. Taking the man by the shoulders he shook open his startled eyes.

'Do you know where the Minnehaha is anchored, and the Privateer?'

As they slid out into the bay he lay back in the stern and stared with vague discontent at the Riviera moon. That was the right moon, all right. Frequently, five nights out of seven, there was the right moon. And here was the soft air, aching with enchantment, and here was the music, many strains of music from many orchestras, drifting out from the shore. Eastward lay the dark Cape of Antibes, and then Nice, and beyond that Monte Carlo, where the night rang chinking full of gold. Some day he would enjoy all that, too, know its every pleasure and success – when he was too old and wise to care.

But tonight – tonight, that stream of silver that waved like a wide strand of curly hair toward the moon; those soft romantic lights of Cannes behind him, the irresistible ineffable love in this air – that was to be wasted forever.

'Which one?' asked the boatman suddenly.

'Which what?' demanded Val, sitting up.

'Which boat?'

He pointed. Val turned; above hovered the grey, sword-like prow of a yacht. During the sustained longing of his wish they had covered half a mile.

He read the brass letters over his head. It was the Privateer, but there were only dim lights on board, and no music and no voices, only a murmurous k-plash at intervals as the small waves leaped at the sides.

'The other one,' said Val; 'the Minnehaha.'

'Don't go yet.'

Val started. The voice, low and soft, had dropped down from the darkness overhead.

'What's the hurry?' said the soft voice. 'Thought maybe somebody was coming to see me, and have suffered terrible disappointment.'

The boatman lifted his oars and looked hesitatingly at Val. But Val was silent, so the man let the blades fall into the water and swept the boat out into the moonlight.

'Wait a minute!' cried Val sharply.

'Good-by,' said the voice. 'Come again when you can stay longer.'

'But I am going to stay now,' he answered breathlessly.

He gave the necessary order and the rowboat swung back to the foot of the small companionway. Someone young, someone in a misty white dress, someone with a lovely low voice, had actually called to him out of the velvet dark. 'If she has eyes!' Val murmured to himself. He liked the romantic sound of it and repeated it under his breath – 'If she has eyes.'

'What are you?' She was directly above him now; she was looking down and he was looking up as he climbed the ladder, and as their eyes met they both began to laugh.

She was very young, slim, almost frail, with a dress that accentuated her youth by its blanched simplicity. Two wan dark spots on her cheeks marked where the colour was by day.

'What are you?' she repeated, moving back and laughing again as his head appeared on the level of the deck. 'I'm frightened now and I want to know.'

'I am a gentleman,' said Val, bowing.

'What sort of a gentleman? There are all sorts of gentlemen.' She broke off. 'You're not American, are you?'

'I'm Russian,' he said, as he might have announced himself to be an archangel. He thought quickly and then added, 'And I am the most fortunate of Russians. All this day, all this spring I have dreamed of falling in love on such a night, and now I see that heaven has sent me to you.'

'Just one moment!' she said, with a little gasp. 'I'm sure now that this visit is a mistake. I don't go in for anything like that. Please!'

'I beg your pardon.' He looked at her in bewilderment, unaware that he had taken too much for granted. Then he drew himself up formally.

'I have made an error. If you will excuse me I will say goodnight.'

He turned away. His hand was on the rail.

'Don't go,' she said, pushing a strand of indefinite hair out of her eyes. 'On second thoughts you can talk any nonsense you like if you'll only not go. I'm miserable and I don't want to be left alone.'

Val hesitated; there was some element in this that he failed to understand. He had taken it for granted that a girl who called to a strange man at night, even from the deck of a yacht, was certainly in a mood for romance. And he wanted intensely to stay. Then he remembered that this was one of the two yachts he had been seeking.

'I imagine that the dinner's on the other boat,' he said.

'The dinner? Oh, yes, it's on the Minnehaha. Were you going there?'

'I was going there – a long time ago.'

'What's your name?'

He was on the point of telling her when something made him ask a question instead.

'And you? Why are you not at the party?'

'Because I preferred to stay here. Mrs Jackson said there would be some Russians there – I suppose that's you.' She looked at him with interest. 'You're a very young man, aren't you?'

'I am much older than I look,' said Val stiffly. 'People always comment on it. It's considered rather a remarkable thing.'

'How old are you?'

'Twenty-one,' he lied.

She laughed.

'What nonsense! You're not more than nineteen.'

His annoyance was so perceptible that she hastened to reassure him. 'Cheer up! I'm only seventeen myself. I might have gone to the party if I'd thought there'd be anyone under fifty there.'

He welcomed the change of subject.

'You preferred to sit and dream here beneath the moon.'

'I've been thinking of mistakes.' They sat down side by side in two canvas deck chairs. 'It's a most engrossing subject – the subject of mistakes. Women very seldom brood about mistakes – they're much more willing to forget than men are. But when they do brood—'

'You have made a mistake?' inquired Val.

She nodded.

'Is it something that cannot be repaired?'

'I think so,' she answered. 'I can't be sure. That's what I was considering when you came along.'

'Perhaps I can help in some way,' said Val. 'Perhaps your mistake is not irreparable, after all.'

'You can't,' she said unhappily. 'So let's not think about it. I'm very tired of my mistake and I'd much rather you'd tell me about all the wonderful, cheerful things that are going on in Cannes tonight.'

They glanced shoreward at the line of mysterious and alluring lights, the big toy banks with candles inside that were really the great fashionable hotels, the lighted clock in the old town, the blurred glow of the Café de Paris, the pricked-out points of villa windows rising on slow hills toward the dark sky.

'What is everyone doing there?' she whispered. 'It looks as though something gorgeous was going on, but what it is I can't quite tell.'

'Everyone there is making love,' said Val quietly.

'Is that it?' She looked for a long time, with a strange expression in her eyes. 'Then I want to go home to America,' she said. 'There is too much love here. I want to go home tomorrow.'

'You are afraid of being in love then?'

She shook her head.

'It isn't that. It's just because – there is no love here for me.'

'Or for me either,' added Val quietly. 'It is sad that we two should be at such a lovely place on such a lovely night and have – nothing.'

He was leaning toward her intently, with a sort of inspired and chaste romance in his eyes – and she drew back.

'Tell me more about yourself,' she inquired quickly. 'If you are Russian where did you learn to speak such excellent English?'

'My mother was American,' he admitted. 'My grandfather was American also, so she had no choice in the matter.'

'Then you're American too!'

'I am Russian,' said Val with dignity.

She looked at him closely, smiled and decided not to argue. 'Well then,' she said diplomatically, 'I suppose you must have a Russian name.'

But he had no intention now of telling her his name. A name, even the Rostoff name, would be a desecration of the night. They were their own low voices, their two faces – and that was enough. He was sure, without any reason for being sure but with a sort of instinct that sang triumphantly through his mind, that in a little while, a minute or an hour, he was going to undergo an initiation into the life of romance. His name had no reality beside what was stirring in his heart.

'You are beautiful,' he said suddenly.

'How do you know?'

'Because for women moonlight is the hardest light of all.'

'Am I nice in the moonlight?'

'You are the loveliest thing that I have ever known.'

'Oh.' She thought this over. 'Of course I had no business to let you come on board. I might have known what we'd talk about – in this moon. But I can't sit here and look at the shore – forever. I'm too young for that. Don't you think I'm too young for that?'

'Much too young,' he agreed solemnly.

Suddenly they both became aware of new music that was close at hand, music that seemed to come out of the water not a hundred yards away.

'Listen!' she cried. 'It's from the Minnehaha. They've finished dinner.'

For a moment they listened in silence.

'Thank you,' said Val suddenly.

'For what?'

He hardly knew he had spoken. He was thanking the deep low horns for singing in the breeze, the sea for its warm murmurous complaint against the bow, the milk of the stars for washing over them until he felt buoyed up in a substance more taut than air.

'So lovely,' she whispered.

'What are we going to do about it?'

'Do we have to do something about it? I thought we could just sit and enjoy—'

'You didn't think that,' he interrupted quietly. 'You know that we must do something about it. I am going to woo you – and you are going to be glad.'

'I can't,' she said very low. She wanted to laugh now, to make some light cool remark that would bring the situation back into the safe waters of a casual flirtation. But it was too late now. Val knew that the music had completed what the moon had begun.

'I will tell you the truth,' he said. 'You are my first love. I am seventeen – the same age as you, no more.'

There was something utterly disarming about the fact that they were the same age. It made her helpless before the fate that had thrown them together. The deck chairs creaked and he was conscious of a faint illusive perfume as they swayed suddenly and childishly together.

III

Whether he kissed her once or several times he could not afterward remember, though it must have been an hour that they sat there close together and he held her hand. What surprised him most about romance was that it seemed to have no element of wild passion – regret, desire, despair – but a delirious promise of such happiness in the world, in living, as he had never known. First love – this was only first love! What must love itself in its fullness, its perfection be.

He did not know that what he was experiencing then, that unreal, undesirous medley of ecstasy and peace, would be unrecapturable forever.

The music had ceased for some time when presently the murmurous silence was broken by the sound of a rowboat disturbing the quiet waves. She sprang suddenly to her feet and her eyes strained out over the bay.

'Listen!' she said quickly. 'I want you to tell me your name.'

'No.'

'Please,' she begged him. 'I'm going away tomorrow.'

He didn't answer.

'I don't want you to forget me,' she said. 'My name is—'

'I won't forget you. I will promise to remember you always. Whoever I may love I will always compare her to you, my first love. So long as I live you will always have that much freshness in my heart.'

'I want you to remember,' she murmured brokenly. 'Oh, this has meant more to me than it has to you – much more.'

She was standing so close to him that he felt her warm young breath on his face. Once again they swayed together. He pressed her hands and wrists between his as it seemed right to do, and kissed her lips. It was the right kiss, he thought, the romantic kiss – not too little or too much. Yet there was a sort of promise in it of other kisses he might have had, and it was with a slight sinking of his heart that he heard the rowboat close to the yacht and realized that her family had returned. The evening was over.

'And this is only the beginning,' he told himself. 'All my life will be like this night.'

She was saying something in a low quick voice and he was listening tensely.

'You must know one thing – I am married. Three months ago.

That was the mistake that I was thinking about when the moon brought you out here. In a moment you will understand.'

She broke off as the boat swung against the companionway and a man's voice floated up out of the darkness.

'Is that you, my dear?'

'Yes.'

'What is this other rowboat waiting?'

'One of Mrs Jackson's guests came here by mistake and I made him stay and amuse me for an hour.'

A moment later the thin white hair and weary face of a man of sixty appeared above the level of the deck. And then Val saw and realized too late how much he cared.

IV

When the Riviera season ended in May the Rostoffs and all the other Russians closed their villas and went north for the summer. The Russian Orthodox Church was locked up and so were the bins of rarer wine, and the fashionable spring moonlight was put away, so to speak, to wait for their return.

'We'll be back next season,' they said as a matter of course.

But this was premature, for they were never coming back any more. Those few who straggled south again after five tragic years were glad to get work as chambermaids or *valets de chambre* in the great hotels where they had once dined. Many of them, of course, were killed in the war or in the revolution; many of them faded out as spongers and small cheats in the big capitals, and not a few ended their lives in a sort of stupefied despair.

When the Kerensky government collapsed in 1917, Val was a lieutenant on the eastern front, trying desperately to enforce authority in his company long after any vestige of it remained. He was still trying when Prince Paul Rostoff and his wife gave up their lives one rainy morning to atone for the blunders of the Romanoffs – and the enviable career of Morris Hasylton's daughter ended in a city that bore even more resemblance to a butcher shop than had Chicago in 1892.

After that Val fought with Denikin's army for a while until he realized that he was participating in a hollow farce and the glory of Imperial Russia was over. Then he went to France and was suddenly confronted with the astounding problem of keeping his body and soul together.

It was, of course, natural that he should think of going to America. Two vague aunts with whom his mother had quarrelled many years ago still lived there in comparative affluence. But the idea was repugnant to the prejudices his mother had implanted in him, and besides he hadn't sufficient money left to pay for his passage over. Until a possible counter-revolution should restore to him the Rostoff properties in Russia he must somehow keep alive in France.

So he went to the little city he knew best of all. He went to Cannes. His last two hundred francs bought him a third-class ticket and when he arrived he gave his dress suit to an obliging party who dealt in such things and received in return money for food and bed. He was sorry afterward that he had sold the dress suit, because it might have helped him to a position as a waiter. But he obtained work as a taxi driver instead and was quite as happy, or rather quite as miserable, at that.

Sometimes he carried Americans to look at villas for rent, and when the front glass of the automobile was up, curious fragments of conversation drifted out to him from within.

'—heard this fellow was a Russian prince.' . . . 'Sh!' . . . 'No, this one right here.' . . . 'Be quiet, Esther!' – followed by subdued laughter.

When the car stopped, his passengers would edge around to

have a look at him. At first he was desperately unhappy when girls did this; after a while he didn't mind any more. Once a cheerfully intoxicated American asked him if it were true and invited him to lunch, and another time an elderly woman seized his hand as she got out of the taxi, shook it violently and then pressed a hundred-franc note into his hand.

'Well, Florence, now I can tell 'em back home I shook hands with a Russian prince.'

The inebriated American who had invited him to lunch thought at first that Val was a son of the czar, and it had to be explained to him that a prince in Russia was simply the equivalent of a British courtesy lord. But he was puzzled that a man of Val's personality didn't go out and make some real money.

'This is Europe,' said Val gravely. 'Here money is not made. It is inherited or else it is slowly saved over a period of many years and maybe in three generations a family moves up into a higher class.'

'Think of something people want – like we do.'

'That is because there is more money to want with in America. Everything that people want here has been thought of long ago.'

But after a year and with the help of a young Englishman he had played tennis with before the war, Val managed to get into the Cannes branch of an English bank. He forwarded mail and bought railroad tickets and arranged tours for impatient sight-seers. Sometimes a familiar face came to his window; if Val was recognized he shook hands; if not he kept silence. After two years he was no longer pointed out as a former prince, for the Russians were an old story now – the splendour of the Rostoffs and their friends was forgotten.

He mixed with people very little. In the evenings he walked for a while on the promenade, took a slow glass of beer in a café and went early to bed. He was seldom invited anywhere because people thought that his sad, intent face was depressing – and he never accepted anyhow. He wore cheap French clothes now instead of the rich tweeds and flannels that had been ordered with his father's from England. As for women, he knew none at all. Of the many things he had been certain about at seventeen, he had been most certain about this – that his life would be full of romance. Now after eight years he knew that it was not to be. Somehow he had never had time for love – the war, the revolution and now his poverty had conspired against his expectant heart. The springs of his emotion which had first poured forth one April night had dried up immediately and only a faint trickle remained.

His happy youth had ended almost before it began. He saw himself growing older and more shabby, and living always more and more in the memories of his gorgeous boyhood. Eventually he would become absurd, pulling out an old heirloom of a watch and showing it to amused young fellow clerks who would listen with winks to his tales of the Rostoff name.

He was thinking these gloomy thoughts one April evening in 1922 as he walked beside the sea and watched the never-changing magic of the awakening lights. It was no longer for his benefit, that magic, but it went on, and he was somehow glad. Tomorrow he was going away on his vacation, to a cheap hotel farther down the shore where he could bathe and rest and read; then he would come back and work some more. Every year for three years he had taken his vacation during the last two weeks in April, perhaps because it was then that he felt the most need for remembering. It was in April that what was destined to be the best part of his life had come to a culmination under a romantic moonlight. It was sacred to him – for what he had thought of as an initiation and a beginning had turned out to be the end.

He paused now in front of the Café des Étrangers and after a moment crossed the street on impulse and sauntered down to the shore. A dozen yachts, already turned to a beautiful silver colour, rode at anchor in the bay. He had seen them that afternoon, and read the names painted on their bows – but only from habit. He had done it for three years now, and it was almost a natural function of his eye.

'*Un beau soir*,' remarked a French voice at his elbow. It was a boatman who had often seen Val here before. 'Monsieur finds the sea beautiful?'

'Very beautiful.'

'I too. But a bad living except in the season. Next week, though, I earn something special. I am paid well for simply waiting here and doing nothing more from eight o'clock until midnight.'

'That's very nice,' said Val politely.

'A widowed lady, very beautiful, from America, whose yacht always anchors in the harbour for the last two weeks in April. If the Privateer comes tomorrow it will make three years.'

V

All night Val didn't sleep – not because there was any question in his mind as to what he should do, but because his long stupefied emotions were suddenly awake and alive. Of course he must not see her – not he, a poor failure with a name that was now only a shadow – but it would make him a little happier always to know that she remembered. It gave his own memory another dimension, raised it like those stereopticon glasses that bring out a picture from the flat paper. It made him sure that he had not deceived himself – he had been charming once upon a time to a lovely woman, and she did not forget.

An hour before train time next day he was at the railway station with his grip, so as to avoid any chance encounter in the street. He found himself a place in a third-class carriage of the waiting train.

Somehow as he sat there he felt differently about life – a sort of hope, faint and illusory, that he hadn't felt twenty-four hours before. Perhaps there was some way in those next few years in which he could make it possible to meet her once again – if he worked hard, threw himself passionately into whatever was at hand. He knew of at least two Russians in Cannes who had started over again with nothing except good manners and ingenuity and were now doing surprisingly well. The blood of Morris Hasylton began to throb a little in Val's temples and made him remember something he had never before cared to remember – that Morris Hasylton, who had built his daughter a palace in St Petersburg, had also started from nothing at all.

Simultaneously another emotion possessed him, less strange, less dynamic but equally American – the emotion of curiosity. In case he did – well, in case life should ever make it possible for him to seek her out, he should at least know her name.

He jumped to his feet, fumbled excitedly at the carriage handle and jumped from the train. Tossing his valise into the check room he started at a run for the American consulate.

'A yacht came in this morning,' he said hurriedly to a clerk, 'an American yacht – the Privateer. I want to know who owns it.'

'Just a minute,' said the clerk, looking at him oddly. 'I'll try to find out.'

After what seemed to Val an interminable time he returned.

'Why, just a minute,' he repeated hesitantly. 'We're – it seems we're finding out.'

'Did the yacht come?'

'Oh, yes – it's here all right. At least I think so. If you'll just wait in that chair.'

After another ten minutes Val looked impatiently at his watch. If they didn't hurry he'd probably miss his train. He made a nervous movement as if to get up from his chair.

'Please sit still,' said the clerk, glancing at him quickly from his desk. 'I ask you. Just sit down in that chair.'

Val stared at him. How could it possibly matter to the clerk whether or not he waited?

'I'll miss my train,' he said impatiently. 'I'm sorry to have given you all this bother—'

'Please sit still! We're glad to get it off our hands. You see, we've been waiting for your inquiry for – ah – three years.'

Val jumped to his feet and jammed his hat on his head.

'Why didn't you tell me that?' he demanded angrily.

'Because we had to get word to our – our client. Please don't go! It's – ah, it's too late.'

Val turned. Someone slim and radiant with dark frightened eyes was standing behind him, framed against the sunshine of the doorway.

'Why—'

Val's lips parted, but no words came through. She took a step toward him.

'I—' She looked at him helplessly, her eyes filling with tears. 'I just wanted to say hello,' she murmured. 'I've come back for three years just because I wanted to say hello.'

Still Val was silent.

'You might answer,' she said impatiently. 'You might answer when I'd – when I'd just about begun to think you'd been killed in the war.' She turned to the clerk. 'Please introduce us!' she cried. 'You see, I can't say hello to him when we don't even know each other's names.'

It's the thing to distrust these international marriages, of course. It's an American tradition that they always turn out badly, and we are accustomed to such headlines as: 'Would Trade Coronet for True American Love, Says Duchess', and 'Claims Count Mendicant Tortured Toledo Wife'. The other sort of headlines are never printed, for who would want to read: 'Castle is Love Nest, Asserts Former Georgia Belle', or 'Duke and Packer's Daughter Celebrate Golden Honeymoon'.

So far there have been no headlines at all about the young Rostoffs. Prince Val is much too absorbed in that string of moonlight-blue taxicabs which he manipulates with such unusual efficiency, to give out interviews. He and his wife only leave New York once a year – but there is still a boatman who rejoices when the Privateer steams into Cannes harbour on a mid-April night.

EVA'S VISIT TO FAIRY-LAND

Louisa May Alcott

Down among the grass and fragrant clover lay little Eva by the brook-side, watching the bright waves, as they went singing by under the drooping flowers that grew on its banks. As she was wondering where the waters went, she heard a faint, low sound, as of far-off music. She thought it was the wind, but not a leaf was stirring, and soon through the rippling water came a strange little boat.

It was a lily of the valley, whose tall stem formed the mast, while the broad leaves that rose from the roots, and drooped again till they reached the water, were filled with little Elves, who danced to the music of the silver lily-bells above, that rang a merry peal, and filled the air with their fragrant breath.

On came the fairy boat, till it reached a moss-grown rock; and here it stopped, while the Fairies rested beneath the violet-leaves, and sang with the dancing waves.

Eva looked with wonder on their gay faces and bright garments, and in the joy of her heart sang too, and threw crimson fruit for the little folks to feast upon.

They looked kindly on the child, and, after whispering long among themselves, two little bright-eyed Elves flew over the shining water, and, lighting on the clover-blossoms, said gently, 'Little maiden, many thanks for your kindness; and our Queen bids us ask if you will go with us to Fairy-Land, and learn what we can teach you.'

'Gladly would I go with you, dear Fairies,' said Eva, 'but I cannot sail in your little boat. See! I can hold you in my hand, and could not live among you without harming your tiny kingdom, I am so large.'

Then the Elves laughed gleefully, as they folded their arms about her, saying, 'You are a good child, dear Eva, to fear doing harm to those weaker than yourself. You cannot hurt us now. Look in the water and see what we have done.'

Eva looked into the brook, and saw a tiny child standing between the Elves. 'Now I can go with you,' said she, 'but see, I can no longer step from the bank to yonder stone, for the brook seems now like a great river, and you have not given me wings like yours.'

But the Fairies took each a hand, and flew lightly over the stream. The Queen and her subjects came to meet her, and all seemed glad to say some kindly word of welcome to the little stranger. They placed a flower-crown upon her head, laid their soft faces against her own, and soon it seemed as if the gentle Elves had always been her friends.

'Now must we go home,' said the Queen, 'and you shall go with us, little one.'

Then there was a great bustle, as they flew about on shining wings, some laying cushions of violet leaves in the boat, others folding the Queen's veil and mantle more closely round her, lest the falling dews should chill her.

The cool waves' gentle plashing against the boat, and the sweet chime of the lily-bells, lulled little Eva to sleep, and when she woke it was in Fairy-Land. A faint, rosy light, as of the setting sun, shone on the white pillars of the Queen's palace as they passed in, and the sleeping flowers leaned gracefully on their stems, dreaming beneath their soft green curtains. All was cool and still, and the Elves glided silently about, lest they should break their slumbers. They led Eva to a bed of pure white leaves, above which drooped the fragrant petals of a crimson rose.

'You can look at the bright colours till the light fades, and then the rose will sing you to sleep,' said the Elves, as they folded the soft leaves about her, gently kissed her and stole away.

Long she lay watching the bright shadows, and listening to the song of the rose, while through the long night dreams of lovely things floated like bright clouds through her mind; while the rose bent lovingly above her, and sang in the clear moonlight.

With the sun rose the Fairies, and, with Eva, hastened away to the fountain, whose cool waters were soon filled with little forms, and the air ringing with happy voices, as the Elves floated in the blue waves among the fair white lilies, or sat on the green moss, smoothing their bright locks, and wearing fresh garlands of dewy flowers. At length the Queen came forth, and her subjects gathered round her, and while the flowers bowed their heads, and the trees hushed their rustling, the Fairies sang their morning hymn to the Father of birds and blossoms, who had made the earth so fair a home for them.

Then they flew away to the gardens, and soon, high up among the tree-tops, or under the broad leaves, sat the Elves in little groups, taking their breakfast of fruit and pure fresh dew; while the bright-winged birds came fearlessly among them, pecking the same ripe berries, and dipping their little beaks in the same flower-cups, and the Fairies folded their arms lovingly about them, smoothed their soft bosoms and joyfully sang to them.

'Now, little Eva,' said they, 'you will see that Fairies are not idle, wilful Spirits, as mortals believe. Come, we will show you what we do.'

They led her to a lovely room, through whose walls of deep green leaves the light stole softly in. Here lay many wounded insects, and harmless little creatures, whom cruel hands had hurt; and pale, drooping flowers grew beside urns of healing herbs, from whose fresh leaves came a faint, sweet perfume.

Eva wondered, but silently followed her guide, little Rose-Leaf, who with tender words passed among the delicate blossoms, pouring dew on their feeble roots, cheering them with her loving words and happy smile.

Then she went to the insects; first to a little fly who lay in a flower-leaf cradle.

'Do you suffer much, dear Gauzy-Wing?' asked the Fairy. 'I will bind up your poor little leg, and Zephyr shall rock you to sleep.' So she folded the cool leaves tenderly about the poor fly, bathed his wings and brought him refreshing drink, while he hummed his thanks, and forgot his pain, as Zephyr softly sung and fanned him with her waving wings.

They passed on, and Eva saw beside each bed a Fairy, who with gentle hands and loving words soothed the suffering insects. At length they stopped beside a bee, who lay among sweet honeysuckle flowers, in a cool, still place, where the summer wind blew in, and the green leaves rustled pleasantly. Yet he seemed to find no rest, and murmured of the pain he was doomed to bear. 'Why must I lie here, while my kindred are out in the pleasant fields, enjoying the sunlight and the fresh air, and cruel hands have doomed me to this dark place and bitter pain when I have done no wrong? Uncared for and forgotten, I must stay here among these poor things who think only of themselves. Come here, Rose-Leaf, and bind up my wounds, for I am far more useful than idle bird or fly.'

Then said the Fairy, while she bathed the broken wing—

'Love-Blossom, you should not murmur. We may find happiness in seeking to be patient even while we suffer. You are not forgotten or uncared for, but others need our care more than you, and to those who take cheerfully the pain and sorrow sent, do we most gladly give our help. You need not be idle, even though lying here in darkness and sorrow; you can be taking from your heart all sad and discontented feelings, and if love and patience blossom there, you will be better for the lonely hours spent here. Look on the bed beside you; this little dove has suffered far greater pain than you, and all our care can never ease it; yet through the long days he hath lain here, not an unkind word or a repining sigh hath he uttered. Ah, Love-Blossom, the gentle bird can teach a lesson you will be wiser and better for.'

Then a faint voice whispered, 'Little Rose-Leaf, come quickly, or I cannot thank you as I ought for all your loving care of me.'

So they passed to the bed beside the discontented bee, and here upon the softest down lay the dove, whose gentle eyes looked gratefully upon the Fairy, as she knelt beside the little couch, smoothed the soft white bosom, folded her arms about it and wept sorrowing tears, while the bird still whispered its gratitude and love.

'Dear Fairy, the fairest flowers have cheered me with their sweet breath, fresh dew and fragrant leaves have been ever ready for me, gentle hands to tend, kindly hearts to love; and for this I can only thank you and say farewell.'

Then the quivering wings were still, and the patient little dove was dead; but the bee murmured no longer, and the dew from the flowers fell like tears around the quiet bed.

Sadly Rose-Leaf led Eva away, saying, 'Lily-Bosom shall have a grave tonight beneath our fairest blossoms, and you shall see that gentleness and love are prized far above gold or beauty, here in Fairy-Land. Come now to the Flower Palace, and see the Fairy Court.'

Beneath green arches, bright with birds and flowers, beside singing waves, went Eva into a lofty hall. The roof of pure white lilies rested on pillars of green clustering vines, while many-coloured blossoms threw their bright shadows on the walls, as they danced below in the deep green moss, and their low, sweet voices sounded softly through the sunlit palace, while the rustling leaves kept time.

Beside the throne stood Eva, and watched the lovely forms around her, as they stood, each little band in its own colour, with glistening wings, and flower wands.

Suddenly the music grew louder and sweeter, and the Fairies knelt, and bowed their heads, as on through the crowd of loving subjects came the Queen, while the air was filled with happy voices singing to welcome her.

She placed the child beside her, saying, 'Little Eva, you shall see now how the flowers on your great earth bloom so brightly. A band of loving little gardeners go daily forth from Fairy-Land, to tend and watch them, that no harm may befall the gentle spirits that dwell beneath their leaves. This is never known, for like all good it is unseen by mortal eyes, and unto only pure hearts like yours do we make known our secret. The humblest flower that grows is visited by our messengers, and often blooms in fragrant beauty unknown, unloved by all save Fairy friends, who seek to fill the spirits with all sweet and gentle virtues, that they may not be useless on the earth; for the noblest mortals stoop to learn of flowers. Now, Eglantine, what have you to tell us of your rosy namesakes on the earth?'

From a group of Elves, whose rose-wreathed wands showed the flower they loved, came one bearing a tiny urn, and, answering the Queen, she said—

'Over hill and valley they are blooming fresh and fair as summer sun and dew can make them. No drooping stem or withered leaf tells of any evil thought within their fragrant bosoms, and thus from the fairest of their race have they gathered this sweet dew, as a token of their gratitude to one whose tenderness and care have kept them pure and happy; and this, the loveliest of their sisters, have I brought to place among the Fairy flowers that never pass away.'

Eglantine laid the urn before the Queen, and placed the fragrant rose on the dewy moss beside the throne, while a murmur of approval went through the hall, as each elfin wand waved to the little Fairy who had toiled so well and faithfully, and could bring so fair a gift to their good Queen.

Then came forth an Elf bearing a withered leaf, while her many-coloured robe and the purple tulips in her hair told her name and charge.

'Dear Queen,' she sadly said, 'I would gladly bring as pleasant tidings as my sister, but, alas! my flowers are proud and wilful, and when I went to gather my little gift of coloured leaves for royal garments, they bade me bring this withered blossom, and tell you they would serve no longer one who will not make them Queen over all the other flowers. They would yield neither dew nor honey, but proudly closed their leaves and bid me go.'

'Your task has been too hard for you,' said the Queen kindly, as she placed the drooping flower in the urn Eglantine had given, 'you will see how this dew from a sweet, pure heart will give new life and loveliness even to this poor faded one. So can you, dear Rainbow, by loving words and gentle teachings, bring back lost purity and peace to those whom pride and selfishness have blighted. Go once again to the proud flowers, and tell them when they are queen of their own hearts they will ask no fairer kingdom. Watch more tenderly than ever over them, see that they lack neither dew nor air, speak lovingly to them, and let no unkind word or deed of theirs anger you. Let them see by your patient love and care how much fairer they might be, and when next you come, you will be laden with gifts from humble, loving flowers.'

Thus they told what they had done, and received from their Queen some gentle chiding or loving word of praise.

'You will be weary of this,' said little Rose-Leaf to Eva; 'come now and see where we are taught to read the tales written on flower-leaves, and the sweet language of the birds, and all that can make a Fairy heart wiser and better.'

Then into a cheerful place they went, where were many groups of flowers, among whose leaves sat the child Elves, and learned from their flower-books all that Fairy hands had written there. Some studied how to watch the tender buds, when to spread them to the sunlight, and when to shelter them from rain; how to guard the ripening seeds, and when to lay them in the warm earth or send them on the summer wind to far off hills and valleys, where other Fairy hands would tend and cherish them, till a sisterhood of happy flowers sprang up to beautify and gladden the lonely spot where they had fallen. Others learned to heal the wounded insects, whose frail limbs a breeze could shatter, and who, were it not for Fairy hands, would die ere half their happy summer life had gone. Some learned how by pleasant dreams to cheer and comfort mortal hearts, by whispered words of love to save from evil deeds those who had gone astray, to fill young hearts with gentle thoughts and pure affections, that no sin might mar the beauty of the human flower; while others, like mortal children, learned the Fairy alphabet. Thus the Elves made loving friends by care and love, and no evil thing could harm them, for those they helped to cherish and protect ever watched to shield and save them.

Eva nodded to the little ones, as they peeped from among the leaves at the stranger, and then she listened to the Fairy lessons. Several tiny Elves stood on a broad leaf while the teacher sat among the petals of a flower that bent beside them, and asked questions that none but Fairies would care to know.

'Twinkle, if there lay nine seeds within a flower-cup and the wind bore five away, how many would the blossom have?' 'Four,' replied the little one.

'Rosebud, if a Cowslip opens three leaves in one day and four the next, how many rosy leaves will there be when the whole flower has bloomed?'

'Seven,' sang the little Elf.

'Harebell, if a silkworm spin one yard of Fairy cloth in an hour, how many will it spin in a day?'

'Twelve,' said the Fairy child.

'Primrose, where lies Violet Island?'

'In the Lake of Ripples.'

'Lilla, you may bound Rose Land.'

'On the north by Ferndale, south by Sunny Wave River, east by the hill of Morning Clouds and west by the Evening Star.'

'Now, little ones,' said the teacher, 'you may go to your painting, that our visitor may see how we repair the flowers that earthly hands have injured.'

Then Eva saw how, on large, white leaves, the Fairies learned to imitate the lovely colours, and with tiny brushes to brighten the blush on the anemone's cheek, to deepen the blue of the violet's eye and add new light to the golden cowslip.

'You have stayed long enough,' said the Elves at length, 'we have many things to show you. Come now and see what is our dearest work.'

So Eva said farewell to the child Elves, and hastened with little Rose-Leaf to the gates. Here she saw many bands of Fairies, folded in dark mantles that mortals might not know them, who, with the child among them, flew away over hill and valley. Some went to the cottages amid the hills, some to the sea-side to watch above the humble fisher folks; but little Rose-Leaf and many others went into the noisy city.

Eva wondered within herself what good the tiny Elves could do in this great place; but she soon learned, for the Fairy band went among the poor and friendless, bringing pleasant dreams to the sick and old, sweet, tender thoughts of love and gentleness to the young, strength to the weak and patient cheerfulness to the poor and lonely.

Then the child wondered no longer, but deeper grew her love for the tender-hearted Elves, who left their own happy home to cheer and comfort those who never knew what hands had clothed and fed them, what hearts had given of their own joy, and brought such happiness to theirs.

Long they stayed, and many a lesson little Eva learned: but when she begged them to go back, they still led her on, saying, 'Our work is not yet done; shall we leave so many sad hearts when we may cheer them, so many dark homes that we may brighten? We must stay yet longer, little Eva, and you may learn yet more.'

Then they went into a dark and lonely room, and here they found a pale, sad-eyed child, who wept bitter tears over a faded flower.

'Ah,' sighed the little one, 'it was my only friend, and I cherished it with all my lone heart's love; 't was all that made my sad life happy; and it is gone.'

Tenderly the child fastened the drooping stem, and placed it where the one faint ray of sunlight stole into the dreary room.

'Do you see,' said the Elves, 'through this simple flower will we keep the child pure and stainless amid the sin and sorrow around her. The love of this shall lead her on through temptation and through grief, and she shall be a spirit of joy and consolation to the sinful and the sorrowing.'

And with busy love toiled the Elves amid the withered leaves, and new strength was given to the flower; while, as day by day the friendless child watered the growing buds, deeper grew her love for the unseen friends who had given her one thing to cherish in her lonely home; sweet, gentle thoughts filled her heart as she bent above it, and the blossom's fragrant breath was to her a whispered voice of all fair and lovely things; and as the flower taught her, so she taught others.

The loving Elves brought her sweet dreams by night, and happy thoughts by day, and as she grew in childlike beauty, pure and patient amid poverty and sorrow, the sinful were rebuked, sorrowing hearts grew light and the weak and selfish forgot their idle fears, when they saw her trustingly live on with none to aid or comfort her. The love she bore the tender flower kept her own heart innocent and bright, and the pure human flower was a lesson to those who looked upon it; and soon the gloomy house was bright with happy hearts, that learned of the gentle child to bear poverty and grief as she had done, to forgive those who brought care and wrong to them, and to seek for happiness in humble deeds of charity and love.

'Our work is done,' whispered the Elves, and with blessings on the two fair flowers, they flew away to other homes – to a blind old man who dwelt alone with none to love him, till through long years of darkness and of silent sorrow the heart within had grown dim and cold. No sunlight could enter at the darkened eyes, and none were near to whisper gentle words, to cheer and comfort.

Thus he dwelt forgotten and alone, seeking to give no joy to others, possessing none himself. Life was dark and sad till the untiring Elves came to his dreary home, bringing sunlight and love. They whispered sweet words of comfort – how, if the darkened eyes could find no light without, within there might be never-failing happiness; gentle feelings and sweet, loving thoughts could make the heart fair, if the gloomy, selfish sorrow were but cast away, and all would be bright and beautiful.

They brought light-hearted children, who gathered round him, making the desolate home fair with their young faces, and his sad heart joyful with their sweet, childish voices. The love they bore he could not cast away, sunlight stole in, the dark thoughts passed away and the earth was a pleasant home to him.

Thus their little hands led him back to peace and happiness, flowers bloomed beside his door, and their fragrant breath brought happy thoughts of pleasant valleys and green hills; birds sang to him, and their sweet voices woke the music in his own soul, that never failed to calm and comfort. Happy sounds were heard in his once lonely home, and bright faces gathered round his knee, and listened tenderly while he strove to tell them all the good that gentleness and love had done for him.

Still the Elves watched near, and brighter grew the heart as kindly thoughts and tender feelings entered in, and made it their home; and when the old man fell asleep, above his grave little feet trod lightly, and loving hands laid fragrant flowers.

Then went the Elves into the dreary prison-houses, where sad hearts pined in lonely sorrow for the joy and freedom they had lost. To these came the loving band with tender words, telling of the peace they yet might win by patient striving and repentant tears, thus waking in their bosoms all the holy feelings and sweet affections that had slept so long.

They told pleasant tales, and sang their sweetest songs to cheer and gladden, while the dim cells grew bright with the sunlight, and fragrant with the flowers the loving Elves had brought, and by their gentle teachings those sad, despairing hearts were filled with patient hope and earnest longing to win back their lost innocence and joy.

Thus to all who needed help or comfort went the faithful Fairies; and when at length they turned towards Fairy-Land, many were the grateful, happy hearts they left behind.

Then through the summer sky, above the blossoming earth, they journeyed home, happier for the joy they had given, wiser for the good they had done.

All Fairy-Land was dressed in flowers, and the soft wind went singing by, laden with their fragrant breath. Sweet music sounded through the air, and troops of Elves in their brightest robes hastened to the palace where the feast was spread.

Soon the bright hall was filled with smiling faces and fair forms, and little Eva, as she stood beside the Queen, thought she had never seen a sight so lovely.

The many-coloured shadows of the fairest flowers played on the pure white walls, and fountains sparkled in the sunlight, making music as the cool waves rose and fell, while to and fro, with waving wings and joyous voices, went the smiling Elves, bearing fruit and honey, or fragrant garlands for each other's hair.

Long they feasted, joyfully they sang, and Eva, dancing merrily among them, longed to be an Elf that she might dwell forever in so fair a home.

At length the music ceased, and the Queen said, as she laid her hand on little Eva's shining hair—

'Dear child, tomorrow we must bear you home, for, much as we long to keep you, it were wrong to bring such sorrow to your loving earthly friends; therefore we will guide you to the brook-side, and there say farewell till you come again to visit us. Nay, do not weep, dear Rose-Leaf; you shall watch over little Eva's flowers, and when she looks at them she will think of you. Come now and lead her to the Fairy garden, and show her what we think our fairest sight. Weep no more, but strive to make her last hours with us happy as you can.'

With gentle caresses and most tender words the loving Elves gathered about the child, and, with Rose-Leaf by her side, they led her through the palace, and along green, winding paths, till Eva saw what seemed a wall of flowers rising before her, while the air was filled with the most fragrant odours, and the low, sweet music as of singing blossoms.

'Where have you brought me, and what mean these lovely sounds?' asked Eva.

'Look here, and you shall see,' said Rose-Leaf, as she bent aside the vines, 'but listen silently or you cannot hear.'

Then Eva, looking through the drooping vines, beheld a garden filled with the loveliest flowers; fair as were all the blossoms she had seen in Fairy-Land, none were so beautiful as these. The rose glowed with a deeper crimson, the lily's soft leaves were more purely white, the crocus and humble cowslip shone like sunlight, and the violet was blue as the sky that smiled above it.

'How beautiful they are,' whispered Eva, 'but, dear Rose-Leaf, why do you keep them here, and why call you this your fairest sight?'

'Look again, and I will tell you,' answered the Fairy.

Eva looked, and saw from every flower a tiny form come forth to welcome the Elves, who all, save Rose-Leaf, had flown above the wall, and were now scattering dew upon the flowers' bright leaves and talking cheerfully with the Spirits, who gathered around them, and seemed full of joy that they had come. The child saw that each one wore the colours of the flower that was its home. Delicate and graceful were the little forms, bright the silken hair that fell about each lovely face; and Eva heard the low, sweet murmur of their silvery voices and the rustle of their wings. She gazed in silent wonder, forgetting she knew not who they were, till the Fairy said—

'These are the spirits of the flowers, and this the Fairy Home where those whose hearts were pure and loving on the earth come to bloom in fadeless beauty here, when their earthly life is past. The humblest flower that blooms has a home with us, for outward beauty is a worthless thing if all be not fair and sweet within. Do you see yonder lovely spirit singing with my sister Moonlight? a clover blossom was her home, and she dwelt unknown, unloved; yet patient and content, bearing cheerfully the sorrows sent her. We watched and saw how fair and sweet the humble flower grew, and then gladly bore her here, to blossom with the lily and the rose. The flowers' lives are often short, for cruel hands destroy them; therefore is it our greatest joy to bring them hither, where no careless foot or wintry wind can harm them, where they bloom in quiet beauty, repaying our care by their love and sweetest perfumes.'

'I will never break another flower,' cried Eva; 'but let me go to them, dear Fairy; I would gladly know the lovely spirits, and ask forgiveness for the sorrow I have caused. May I not go in?'

'Nay, dear Eva, you are a mortal child, and cannot enter here; but I will tell them of the kind little maiden who has learned to love them, and they will remember you when you are gone. Come now, for you have seen enough, and we must be away.'

On a rosy morning cloud, surrounded by the loving Elves, went Eva through the sunny sky. The fresh wind bore them gently on, and soon they stood again beside the brook, whose waves danced brightly as if to welcome them.

'Now, ere we say farewell,' said the Queen, as they gathered nearer to the child, 'tell me, dear Eva, what among all our Fairy gifts will make you happiest, and it shall be yours.'

'You good little Fairies,' said Eva, folding them in her arms, for she was no longer the tiny child she had been in Fairy-Land, 'you dear good little Elves, what can I ask of you, who have done so much to make me happy, and taught me so many good and gentle lessons, the memory of which will never pass away? I can only ask of you the power to be as pure and gentle as yourselves, as tender and loving to the weak and sorrowing, as untiring in kindly deeds to all. Grant me this gift, and you shall see that little Eva has not forgotten what you have taught her.'

'The power shall be yours,' said the Elves, and laid their soft hands on her head; 'we will watch over you in dreams, and when you would have tidings of us, ask the flowers in your garden, and they will tell you all you would know. Farewell. Remember Fairy-Land and all your loving friends.'

They clung about her tenderly, and little Rose-Leaf placed a flower crown on her head, whispering softly, 'When you would come to us again, stand by the brook-side and wave this in the air, and we will gladly take you to our home again. Farewell, dear Eva. Think of your little Rose-Leaf when among the flowers.'

Long Eva watched their shining wings, and listened to the music of their voices as they flew singing home, and when at length the last little form had vanished among the clouds, she saw that all around her where the Elves had been, the fairest flowers had sprung up, and the lonely brook-side was a blooming garden.

Thus she stood among the waving blossoms, with the Fairy garland in her hair, and happy feelings in her heart, better and wiser for her visit to Fairy-Land.

THE ADVENTURE OF THE BLUE CARBUNCLE

Arthur Conan Doyle

I had called upon my friend Sherlock Holmes upon the second morning after Christmas, with the intention of wishing him the compliments of the season. He was lounging upon the sofa in a purple dressing-gown, a pipe-rack within his reach upon the right, and a pile of crumpled morning papers, evidently newly studied, near at hand. Beside the couch was a wooden chair, and on the angle of the back hung a very seedy and disreputable hard-felt hat, much the worse for wear, and cracked in several places. A lens and a forceps lying upon the seat of the chair suggested that the hat had been suspended in this manner for the purpose of examination.

'You are engaged,' said I; 'perhaps I interrupt you.'

'Not at all. I am glad to have a friend with whom I can discuss my results. The matter is a perfectly trivial one' – he jerked his thumb in the direction of the old hat – 'but there are points in connection with it which are not entirely devoid of interest and even of instruction.'

I seated myself in his armchair and warmed my hands before his crackling fire, for a sharp frost had set in, and the windows were thick with the ice crystals. 'I suppose,' I remarked, 'that, homely as it looks, this thing has some deadly story linked on to it – that it is the clue which will guide you in the solution of some mystery and the punishment of some crime.'

'No, no. No crime,' said Sherlock Holmes, laughing. 'Only one of those whimsical little incidents which will happen when you have four million human beings all jostling each other within the space of a few square miles. Amid the action and reaction of so dense a swarm of humanity, every possible combination of events may be expected to take place, and many a little problem will be presented which may be striking and bizarre without being criminal. We have already had experience of such.'

'So much so,' I remarked, 'that of the last six cases which I have added to my notes, three have been entirely free of any legal crime.'

'Precisely. You allude to my attempt to recover the Irene Adler papers, to the singular case of Miss Mary Sutherland and to the adventure of the man with the twisted lip. Well, I have no doubt that this small matter will fall into the same innocent category. You know Peterson, the commissionaire?'

'Yes.'

'It is to him that this trophy belongs.'

'It is his hat.'

'No, no, he found it. Its owner is unknown. I beg that you will look upon it not as a battered billycock but as an intellectual problem. And, first, as to how it came here. It arrived upon Christmas morning, in company with a good fat goose, which is, I have no doubt, roasting at this moment in front of Peterson's fire. The facts are these: about four o'clock on Christmas morning, Peterson, who, as you know, is a very honest fellow, was returning from some small jollification and was making his way homeward down Tottenham Court Road. In front of him he saw, in the gaslight, a tallish man, walking with a slight stagger, and carrying a white goose slung over his shoulder. As he reached the corner of Goodge Street, a row broke out between this stranger and a little knot of roughs. One of the latter knocked off the man's hat, on which he raised his stick to defend himself and, swinging it over his head, smashed the shop window behind him. Peterson had rushed forward to protect the stranger from his assailants; but the man, shocked at having broken the window, and seeing an official-looking person in uniform rushing towards him, dropped his goose, took to his heels and vanished amid the labyrinth of small streets which lie at the back of Tottenham Court Road. The roughs had also fled at the appearance of Peterson, so that he was left in possession of the field of battle, and also of the spoils of victory in the shape of this battered hat and a most unimpeachable Christmas goose.'

'Which surely he restored to their owner?'

'My dear fellow, there lies the problem. It is true that "For Mrs Henry Baker" was printed upon a small card which was tied to the bird's left leg, and it is also true that the initials "H B" are legible upon the lining of this hat, but as there are some thousands of Bakers, and some hundreds of Henry Bakers in this city of ours, it is not easy to restore lost property to any one of them.'

'What, then, did Peterson do?'

'He brought round both hat and goose to me on Christmas morning, knowing that even the smallest problems are of interest to me. The goose we retained until this morning, when there were signs that, in spite of the slight frost, it would be well that it should be eaten without unnecessary delay. Its finder has carried it off, therefore, to fulfil the ultimate destiny of a goose, while I continue to retain the hat of the unknown gentleman who lost his Christmas dinner.'

'Did he not advertise?'

'No.'

'Then, what clue could you have as to his identity?'

'Only as much as we can deduce.'

'From his hat?'

'Precisely.'

'But you are joking. What can you gather from this old battered felt?'

'Here is my lens. You know my methods. What can you gather yourself as to the individuality of the man who has worn this article?'

I took the tattered object in my hands and turned it over rather ruefully. It was a very ordinary black hat of the usual round shape, hard and much the worse for wear. The lining had been of red silk, but was a good deal discoloured. There was no maker's name; but, as Holmes had remarked, the initials 'H B' were scrawled upon one side. It was pierced in the brim for a hat-securer, but the elastic was missing. For the rest, it was cracked, exceedingly dusty and spotted in several places, although there seemed to have been some attempt to hide the discoloured patches by smearing them with ink.

'I can see nothing,' said I, handing it back to my friend.

'On the contrary, Watson, you can see everything. You fail, however, to reason from what you see. You are too timid in drawing your inferences.'

'Then, pray tell me what it is that you can infer from this hat?'

He picked it up and gazed at it in the peculiar introspective fashion which was characteristic of him. 'It is perhaps less suggestive than it might have been,' he remarked, 'and yet there are a few inferences which are very distinct, and a few others which represent at least a strong balance of probability. That the man was highly intellectual is of course obvious upon the face of it, and also that he was fairly well-to-do within the last three years, although he has now fallen upon evil days. He had foresight, but has less now than formerly, pointing to a moral retrogression, which, when taken with the decline of his fortunes, seems to indicate some evil influence, probably drink, at work upon him. This may account also for the obvious fact that his wife has ceased to love him.'

'My dear Holmes!'

'He has, however, retained some degree of self-respect,' he continued, disregarding my remonstrance. 'He is a man who leads a sedentary life, goes out little, is out of training entirely, is middle-aged, has grizzled hair which he has had cut within the last few days and which he anoints with lime-cream. These are the more patent facts which are to be deduced from his hat. Also, by the way, that it is extremely improbable that he has gas laid on in his house.'

'You are certainly joking, Holmes.'

'Not in the least. Is it possible that even now, when I give you these results, you are unable to see how they are attained?'

'I have no doubt that I am very stupid, but I must confess that I am unable to follow you. For example, how did you deduce that this man was intellectual?'

For answer Holmes clapped the hat upon his head. It came right over the forehead and settled upon the bridge of his nose. 'It is a question of cubic capacity,' said he; 'a man with so large a brain must have something in it.'

'The decline of his fortunes, then?'

'This hat is three years old. These flat brims curled at the edge came in then. It is a hat of the very best quality. Look at the band of ribbed silk and the excellent lining. If this man could afford to buy so expensive a hat three years ago, and has had no hat since, then he has assuredly gone down in the world.'

'Well, that is clear enough, certainly. But how about the foresight and the moral retrogression?'

Sherlock Holmes laughed. 'Here is the foresight,' said he putting his finger upon the little disc and loop of the hat-securer. 'They are never sold upon hats. If this man ordered one, it is a sign of a certain amount of foresight, since he went out of his way to take this precaution against the wind. But since we see that he has broken the elastic and has not troubled to replace it, it is obvious that he has less foresight now than formerly, which is a distinct proof of a weakening nature. On the other hand, he has endeavoured to conceal some of these stains upon the felt by daubing them with ink, which is a sign that he has not entirely lost his self-respect.'

'Your reasoning is certainly plausible.'

'The further points, that he is middle-aged, that his hair is grizzled, that it has been recently cut and that he uses lime-cream, are all to be gathered from a close examination of the lower part of the lining. The lens discloses a large number of hair-ends, clean cut by the scissors of the barber. They all appear to be adhesive, and there is a distinct odour of lime-cream. This dust, you will observe, is not the gritty, grey dust of the street but the fluffy brown dust of the house, showing that it has been hung up indoors most of the time, while the marks of moisture upon the inside are proof positive that the wearer perspired very freely, and could therefore, hardly be in the best of training.'

'But his wife – you said that she had ceased to love him.'

'This hat has not been brushed for weeks. When I see you, my dear Watson, with a week's accumulation of dust upon your hat, and when your wife allows you to go out in such a state, I shall fear that you also have been unfortunate enough to lose your wife's affection.'

'But he might be a bachelor.'

'Nay, he was bringing home the goose as a peace-offering to his wife. Remember the card upon the bird's leg.'

'You have an answer to everything. But how on earth do you deduce that the gas is not laid on in his house?'

'One tallow stain, or even two, might come by chance; but when

I see no less than five, I think that there can be little doubt that the individual must be brought into frequent contact with burning tallow – walks upstairs at night probably with his hat in one hand and a guttering candle in the other. Anyhow, he never got tallow-stains from a gas-jet. Are you satisfied?'

'Well, it is very ingenious,' said I, laughing; 'but since, as you said just now, there has been no crime committed, and no harm done save the loss of a goose, all this seems to be rather a waste of energy.'

Sherlock Holmes had opened his mouth to reply, when the door flew open, and Peterson, the commissionaire, rushed into the apartment with flushed cheeks and the face of a man who is dazed with astonishment.

'The goose, Mr Holmes! The goose, sir!' he gasped.

'Eh? What of it, then? Has it returned to life and flapped off through the kitchen window?' Holmes twisted himself round upon the sofa to get a fairer view of the man's excited face.

'See here, sir! See what my wife found in its crop!' He held out his hand and displayed upon the centre of the palm a brilliantly scintillating blue stone, rather smaller than a bean in size, but of such purity and radiance that it twinkled like an electric point in the dark hollow of his hand.

Sherlock Holmes sat up with a whistle. 'By Jove, Peterson!' said he, 'this is treasure trove indeed. I suppose you know what you have got?'

'A diamond, sir? A precious stone. It cuts into glass as though it were putty.'

'It's more than a precious stone. It is *the* precious stone.'

'Not the Countess of Morcar's blue carbuncle!' I ejaculated.

'Precisely so. I ought to know its size and shape, seeing that I have read the advertisement about it in *The Times* every day lately. It is absolutely unique, and its value can only be conjectured, but the reward offered of £1000 is certainly not within a twentieth part of the market price.'

'A thousand pounds! Great Lord of mercy!' The commissionaire plumped down into a chair and stared from one to the other of us.

'That is the reward, and I have reason to know that there are sentimental considerations in the background which would induce the Countess to part with half her fortune if she could but recover the gem.'

'It was lost, if I remember aright, at the Hotel Cosmopolitan,' I remarked.

'Precisely so, on December 22nd, just five days ago. John Horner, a plumber, was accused of having abstracted it from the lady's jewel-case. The evidence against him was so strong that the case has been referred to the Assizes. I have some account of the matter here, I believe.' He rummaged amid his newspapers, glancing over the dates, until at last he smoothed one out, doubled it over and read the following paragraph:

'Hotel Cosmopolitan Jewel Robbery. John Horner, 26, plumber, was brought up upon the charge of having upon the 22nd inst., abstracted from the jewel-case of the Countess of Morcar the valuable gem known as the blue carbuncle. James Ryder, upper-attendant at the hotel, gave his evidence to the effect that he had shown Horner up to the dressing-room of the Countess of Morcar upon the day of the robbery in order that he might solder the second bar of the grate, which was loose. He had remained with Horner some little time, but had finally been called away. On returning, he found that Horner had disappeared, that the bureau had been forced open and that the small morocco casket in which, as it afterwards transpired, the Countess was accustomed to keep her jewel, was lying empty upon the dressing-table. Ryder instantly gave the alarm, and Horner was arrested the same evening; but the stone could not be found either upon his person or in his rooms. Catherine Cusack, maid to the Countess, deposed to having heard Ryder's cry of dismay on discovering the robbery, and to having rushed into the room, where she found matters as described by the last witness. Inspector Bradstreet, B division, gave evidence as to the arrest of Horner, who struggled frantically, and protested his innocence in the strongest terms. Evidence of a previous conviction for robbery having been given against the prisoner, the magistrate refused to deal summarily with the offence, but referred it to the Assizes. Horner, who had shown signs of intense emotion during the proceedings, fainted away at the conclusion and was carried out of court.'

'Hum! So much for the police-court,' said Holmes thoughtfully, tossing aside the paper. 'The question for us now to solve is the sequence of events leading from a rifled jewel-case at one end to the crop of a goose in Tottenham Court Road at the other. You see, Watson, our little deductions have suddenly assumed a much more important and less innocent aspect. Here is the stone; the stone came from the goose, and the goose came from Mr Henry Baker, the gentleman with the bad hat and all the other characteristics with which I have bored you. So now we must set ourselves very seriously to finding this gentleman and ascertaining what part he has played in this little mystery. To do this, we must try the simplest means first, and these lie undoubtedly in an advertisement in all the evening papers. If this fail, I shall have recourse to other methods.'

'What will you say?'

'Give me a pencil and that slip of paper. Now, then: "Found at the corner of Goodge Street, a goose and a black felt hat. Mr Henry Baker can have the same by applying at 6:30 this evening at 221B, Baker Street." That is clear and concise.'

'Very. But will he see it?'

'Well, he is sure to keep an eye on the papers, since, to a poor man, the loss was a heavy one. He was clearly so scared by his mischance in breaking the window and by the approach of Peterson that he thought of nothing but flight, but since then he must have bitterly regretted the impulse which caused him to drop his bird. Then, again, the introduction of his name will cause him to see it, for everyone who knows him will direct his attention to it. Here you are, Peterson, run down to the advertising agency and have this put in the evening papers.'

'In which, sir?'

'Oh, in the *Globe*, *Star*, *Pall Mall*, *St James's Gazette*, *Evening News*, *Standard*, *Echo* and any others that occur to you.'

'Very well, sir. And this stone?'

'Ah, yes, I shall keep the stone. Thank you. And, I say, Peterson, just buy a goose on your way back and leave it here with me, for we must have one to give to this gentleman in place of the one which your family is now devouring.'

When the commissionaire had gone, Holmes took up the stone and held it against the light. 'It's a bonny thing,' said he. 'Just see how it glints and sparkles. Of course it is a nucleus and focus of crime. Every good stone is. They are the devil's pet baits. In the larger and older jewels every facet may stand for a bloody deed. This stone is not yet twenty years old. It was found in the banks of the Amoy River in southern China and is remarkable in having every characteristic of the carbuncle, save that it is blue in shade instead of ruby red. In spite of its youth, it has already a sinister history. There have been two murders, a vitriol-throwing, a suicide and several robberies brought about for the sake of this forty-grain weight of crystallized charcoal. Who would think that so pretty a toy would be a purveyor to the gallows and the prison? I'll lock it up in my strong box now and drop a line to the Countess to say that we have it.'

'Do you think that this man Horner is innocent?'

'I cannot tell.'

'Well, then, do you imagine that this other one, Henry Baker, had anything to do with the matter?'

'It is, I think, much more likely that Henry Baker is an absolutely innocent man, who had no idea that the bird which he was carrying was of considerably more value than if it were made of solid gold. That, however, I shall determine by a very simple test if we have an answer to our advertisement.'

'And you can do nothing until then?'

'Nothing.'

'In that case I shall continue my professional round. But I shall come back in the evening at the hour you have mentioned, for I should like to see the solution of so tangled a business.'

'Very glad to see you. I dine at seven. There is a woodcock, I believe. By the way, in view of recent occurrences, perhaps I ought to ask Mrs Hudson to examine its crop.'

I had been delayed at a case, and it was a little after half-past six when I found myself in Baker Street once more. As I approached the house I saw a tall man in a Scotch bonnet with a coat which was buttoned up to his chin waiting outside in the bright semicircle which was thrown from the fanlight. Just as I arrived the door was opened, and we were shown up together to Holmes' room.

'Mr Henry Baker, I believe,' said he, rising from his armchair and greeting his visitor with the easy air of geniality which he could so readily assume. 'Pray take this chair by the fire, Mr Baker. It is a cold night, and I observe that your circulation is more adapted for summer than for winter. Ah, Watson, you have just come at the right time. Is that your hat, Mr Baker?'

'Yes, sir, that is undoubtedly my hat.'

He was a large man with rounded shoulders, a massive head and a broad, intelligent face, sloping down to a pointed beard of grizzled brown. A touch of red in nose and cheeks, with a slight tremor of his extended hand, recalled Holmes' surmise as to his habits. His rusty black frock-coat was buttoned right up in front, with the collar turned up, and his lank wrists protruded from his sleeves without a sign of cuff or shirt. He spoke in a slow staccato fashion, choosing his words with care, and gave the impression generally of a man of learning and letters who had had ill-usage at the hands of fortune.

'We have retained these things for some days,' said Holmes, 'because we expected to see an advertisement from you giving your address. I am at a loss to know now why you did not advertise.'

Our visitor gave a rather shamefaced laugh. 'Shillings have not been so plentiful with me as they once were,' he remarked. 'I had no doubt that the gang of roughs who assaulted me had carried off both my hat and the bird. I did not care to spend more money in a hopeless attempt at recovering them.'

'Very naturally. By the way, about the bird, we were compelled to eat it.'

'To eat it!' Our visitor half rose from his chair in his excitement.

'Yes, it would have been of no use to anyone had we not done so. But I presume that this other goose upon the sideboard, which is about the same weight and perfectly fresh, will answer your purpose equally well?'

'Oh, certainly, certainly,' answered Mr Baker with a sigh of relief.

'Of course, we still have the feathers, legs, crop and so on of your own bird, so if you wish—'

The man burst into a hearty laugh. 'They might be useful to me as relics of my adventure,' said he, 'but beyond that I can hardly see what use the *disjecta membra* of my late acquaintance are going to be to me. No, sir, I think that, with your permission, I will confine my attentions to the excellent bird which I perceive upon the sideboard.'

Sherlock Holmes glanced sharply across at me with a slight shrug of his shoulders.

'There is your hat, then, and there your bird,' said he. 'By the way, would it bore you to tell me where you got the other one from? I am somewhat of a fowl fancier, and I have seldom seen a better grown goose.'

'Certainly, sir,' said Baker, who had risen and tucked his newly gained property under his arm. 'There are a few of us who frequent the Alpha Inn, near the Museum – we are to be found in the Museum itself during the day, you understand. This year our good host, Windigate by name, instituted a goose club, by which, on consideration of some few pence every week, we were each to receive a bird at Christmas. My pence were duly paid, and the rest is familiar to you. I am much indebted to you, sir, for a Scotch bonnet is fitted neither to my years nor my gravity.' With a comical pomposity of manner he bowed solemnly to both of us and strode off upon his way.

'So much for Mr Henry Baker,' said Holmes when he had closed the door behind him. 'It is quite certain that he knows nothing whatever about the matter. Are you hungry, Watson?'

'Not particularly.'

'Then I suggest that we turn our dinner into a supper and follow up this clue while it is still hot.'

'By all means.'

It was a bitter night, so we drew on our ulsters and wrapped cravats about our throats. Outside, the stars were shining coldly in a cloudless sky, and the breath of the passers-by blew out into smoke like so many pistol shots. Our footfalls rang out crisply and loudly as we swung through the doctors' quarter, Wimpole Street, Harley Street, and so through Wigmore Street into Oxford Street. In a quarter of an hour we were in Bloomsbury at the Alpha Inn, which is a small public-house at the corner of one of the streets which runs down into Holborn. Holmes pushed open the door of the private bar and ordered two glasses of beer from the ruddy-faced, white-aproned landlord.

'Your beer should be excellent if it is as good as your geese,' said he.

'My geese!' The man seemed surprised.

'Yes. I was speaking only half an hour ago to Mr Henry Baker, who was a member of your goose club.'

'Ah! yes, I see. But you see, sir, them's not *our* geese.'

'Indeed! Whose, then?'

'Well, I got the two dozen from a salesman in Covent Garden.'

'Indeed? I know some of them. Which was it?'

'Breckinridge is his name.'

'Ah! I don't know him. Well, here's your good health, landlord, and prosperity to your house. Good-night.'

'Now for Mr Breckinridge,' he continued, buttoning up his coat as we came out into the frosty air. 'Remember, Watson, that though we have so homely a thing as a goose at one end of this chain, we have at the other a man who will certainly get seven years' penal servitude unless we can establish his innocence. It is possible that our inquiry may but confirm his guilt; but, in any case, we have a line of investigation which has been missed by the police, and which a singular chance has placed in our hands. Let us follow it out to the bitter end. Faces to the south, then, and quick march!'

We passed across Holborn, down Endell Street, and so through a zigzag of slums to Covent Garden Market. One of the largest stalls bore the name of Breckinridge upon it, and the proprietor, a horsey-looking man, with a sharp face and trim side-whiskers, was helping a boy to put up the shutters.

'Good-evening. It's a cold night,' said Holmes.

The salesman nodded and shot a questioning glance at my companion.

'Sold out of geese, I see,' continued Holmes, pointing at the bare slabs of marble.

'Let you have five hundred to-morrow morning.'

'That's no good.'

'Well, there are some on the stall with the gas-flare.'

'Ah, but I was recommended to you.'

'Who by?'

'The landlord of the Alpha.'

'Oh, yes; I sent him a couple of dozen.'

'Fine birds they were, too. Now where did you get them from?'

To my surprise the question provoked a burst of anger from the salesman.

'Now, then, mister,' said he, with his head cocked and his arms akimbo, 'what are you driving at? Let's have it straight, now.'

'It is straight enough. I should like to know who sold you the geese which you supplied to the Alpha.'

'Well then, I shan't tell you. So now!'

'Oh, it is a matter of no importance; but I don't know why you should be so warm over such a trifle.'

'Warm! You'd be as warm, maybe, if you were as pestered as I am. When I pay good money for a good article there should be an end of the business; but it's "Where are the geese?" and "Who did you sell the geese to?" and "What will you take for the geese?" One would think they were the only geese in the world, to hear the fuss that is made over them.'

'Well, I have no connection with any other people who have been making inquiries,' said Holmes carelessly. 'If you won't tell us the bet is off, that is all. But I'm always ready to back my opinion on a matter of fowls, and I have a fiver on it that the bird I ate is country bred.'

'Well, then, you've lost your fiver, for it's town bred,' snapped the salesman.

'It's nothing of the kind.'

'I say it is.'

'I don't believe it.'

'D'you think you know more about fowls than I, who have handled them ever since I was a nipper? I tell you, all those birds that went to the Alpha were town bred.'

'You'll never persuade me to believe that.'

'Will you bet, then?'

'It's merely taking your money, for I know that I am right. But I'll have a sovereign on with you, just to teach you not to be obstinate.'

The salesman chuckled grimly. 'Bring me the books, Bill,' said he.

The small boy brought round a small thin volume and a great greasy-backed one, laying them out together beneath the hanging lamp.

'Now then, Mr Cocksure,' said the salesman, 'I thought that I was out of geese, but before I finish you'll find that there is still one left in my shop. You see this little book?'

'Well?'

'That's the list of the folk from whom I buy. D'you see? Well, then, here on this page are the country folk, and the numbers after their names are where their accounts are in the big ledger. Now, then! You see this other page in red ink? Well, that is a list of my town suppliers. Now, look at that third name. Just read it out to me.'

'"Mrs Oakshott, 117, Brixton Road – 249,"' read Holmes.

'Quite so. Now turn that up in the ledger.'

Holmes turned to the page indicated. 'Here you are, "Mrs Oakshott, 117, Brixton Road, egg and poultry supplier."'

'Now, then, what's the last entry?'

'"December 22nd. Twenty-four geese at 7s. 6d."'

'Quite so. There you are. And underneath?'

'"Sold to Mr Windigate of the Alpha, at 12s."'

'What have you to say now?'

Sherlock Holmes looked deeply chagrined. He drew a sovereign from his pocket and threw it down upon the slab, turning away with the air of a man whose disgust is too deep for words. A few yards off he stopped under a lamp-post and laughed in the hearty, noiseless fashion which was peculiar to him.

'When you see a man with whiskers of that cut and the "Pink 'un" protruding out of his pocket, you can always draw him by a bet,' said he. 'I daresay that if I had put £100 down in front of him, that man would not have given me such complete information as was drawn from him by the idea that he was doing me on a wager. Well, Watson, we are, I fancy, nearing the end of our quest, and the only point which remains to be determined is whether we should go on to this Mrs Oakshott to-night, or whether we should reserve it for to-morrow. It is clear from what that surly fellow said that there are others besides ourselves who are anxious about the matter, and I should—'

His remarks were suddenly cut short by a loud hubbub which broke out from the stall which we had just left. Turning round we saw a little rat-faced fellow standing in the centre of the circle of yellow light which was thrown by the swinging lamp, while Breckinridge, the salesman, framed in the door of his stall, was shaking his fists fiercely at the cringing figure.

'I've had enough of you and your geese,' he shouted. 'I wish you were all at the devil together. If you come pestering me any more with your silly talk I'll set the dog at you. You bring Mrs Oakshott here and I'll answer her, but what have you to do with it? Did I buy the geese off you?'

'No; but one of them was mine all the same,' whined the little man.

'Well, then, ask Mrs Oakshott for it.'

'She told me to ask you.'

'Well, you can ask the King of Proosia, for all I care. I've had enough of it. Get out of this!' He rushed fiercely forward, and the inquirer flitted away into the darkness.

'Ha! this may save us a visit to Brixton Road,' whispered Holmes. 'Come with me, and we will see what is to be made of this fellow.' Striding through the scattered knots of people who lounged round the flaring stalls, my companion speedily overtook the little man and touched him upon the shoulder. He sprang round, and I could see in the gas-light that every vestige of colour had been driven from his face.

'Who are you, then? What do you want?' he asked in a quavering voice.

'You will excuse me,' said Holmes blandly, 'but I could not help overhearing the questions which you put to the salesman just now. I think that I could be of assistance to you.'

'You? Who are you? How could you know anything of the matter?'

'My name is Sherlock Holmes. It is my business to know what other people don't know.'

'But you can know nothing of this?'

'Excuse me, I know everything of it. You are endeavouring to trace some geese which were sold by Mrs Oakshott, of Brixton Road, to a salesman named Breckinridge, by him in turn to Mr Windigate, of the Alpha, and by him to his club, of which Mr Henry Baker is a member.'

'Oh, sir, you are the very man whom I have longed to meet,' cried the little fellow with outstretched hands and quivering fingers. 'I can hardly explain to you how interested I am in this matter.'

Sherlock Holmes hailed a four-wheeler which was passing. 'In that case we had better discuss it in a cosy room rather than in this wind-swept market-place,' said he. 'But pray tell me, before we go farther, who it is that I have the pleasure of assisting.'

The man hesitated for an instant. 'My name is John Robinson,' he answered with a sidelong glance.

'No, no; the real name,' said Holmes sweetly. 'It is always awkward doing business with an alias.'

A flush sprang to the white cheeks of the stranger. 'Well then,' said he, 'my real name is James Ryder.'

'Precisely so. Head attendant at the Hotel Cosmopolitan. Pray step into the cab, and I shall soon be able to tell you everything which you would wish to know.'

The little man stood glancing from one to the other of us with half-frightened, half-hopeful eyes, as one who is not sure whether he is on the verge of a windfall or of a catastrophe. Then he stepped into the cab, and in half an hour we were back in the sitting-room at Baker Street. Nothing had been said during our drive, but the high, thin breathing of our new companion, and the claspings and unclaspings of his hands, spoke of the nervous tension within him.

'Here we are!' said Holmes cheerily as we filed into the room. 'The fire looks very seasonable in this weather. You look cold, Mr Ryder. Pray take the basket-chair. I will just put on my slippers before we settle this little matter of yours. Now, then! You want to know what became of those geese?'

'Yes, sir.'

'Or rather, I fancy, of that goose. It was one bird, I imagine, in which you were interested – white, with a black bar across the tail.'

Ryder quivered with emotion. 'Oh, sir,' he cried, 'can you tell me where it went to?'

'It came here.'

'Here?'

'Yes, and a most remarkable bird it proved. I don't wonder that you should take an interest in it. It laid an egg after it was dead – the bonniest, brightest little blue egg that ever was seen. I have it here in my museum.'

Our visitor staggered to his feet and clutched the mantelpiece with his right hand. Holmes unlocked his strong-box and held up the blue carbuncle, which shone out like a star, with a cold, brilliant, many-pointed radiance. Ryder stood glaring with a drawn face, uncertain whether to claim or to disown it.

'The game's up, Ryder,' said Holmes quietly. 'Hold up, man, or you'll be into the fire! Give him an arm back into his chair, Watson. He's not got blood enough to go in for felony with impunity. Give him a dash of brandy. So! Now he looks a little more human. What a shrimp it is, to be sure!'

For a moment he had staggered and nearly fallen, but the brandy brought a tinge of colour into his cheeks, and he sat staring with frightened eyes at his accuser.

'I have almost every link in my hands, and all the proofs which I could possibly need, so there is little which you need tell me. Still, that little may as well be cleared up to make the case complete. You had heard, Ryder, of this blue stone of the Countess of Morcar's?'

'It was Catherine Cusack who told me of it,' said he in a crackling voice.

'I see – her ladyship's waiting-maid. Well, the temptation of sudden wealth so easily acquired was too much for you, as it has been for better men before you; but you were not very scrupulous in the means you used. It seems to me, Ryder, that there is the making of a very pretty villain in you. You knew that this man Horner, the plumber, had been concerned in some such matter before, and that suspicion would rest the more readily upon him. What did you do, then? You made some small job in my lady's room – you and your confederate Cusack – and you managed that he should be the man sent for. Then, when he had left, you rifled the jewel-case, raised the alarm and had this unfortunate man arrested. You then—'

Ryder threw himself down suddenly upon the rug and clutched at my companion's knees. 'For God's sake, have mercy!' he shrieked. 'Think of my father! Of my mother! It would break their hearts. I never went wrong before! I never will again. I swear it. I'll swear it on a Bible. Oh, don't bring it into court! For Christ's sake, don't!'

'Get back into your chair!' said Holmes sternly. 'It is very well to cringe and crawl now, but you thought little enough of this poor Horner in the dock for a crime of which he knew nothing.'

'I will fly, Mr Holmes. I will leave the country, sir. Then the charge against him will break down.'

'Hum! We will talk about that. And now let us hear a true account of the next act. How came the stone into the goose, and how came the goose into the open market? Tell us the truth, for there lies your only hope of safety.'

Ryder passed his tongue over his parched lips. 'I will tell you it just as it happened, sir,' said he. 'When Horner had been arrested, it seemed to me that it would be best for me to get away with the stone at once, for I did not know at what moment the police might not take it into their heads to search me and my room. There was no place about the hotel where it would be safe. I went out, as if on some commission, and I made for my sister's house. She had married a man named Oakshott, and lived in Brixton Road, where she fattened fowls for the market. All the way there every man I met seemed to me to be a policeman or a detective; and, for all that it was a cold night, the sweat was pouring down my face before I came to the Brixton Road. My sister asked me what was the matter, and why I was so pale; but I told her that I had been upset by the jewel robbery at the hotel. Then I went into the back yard and smoked a pipe and wondered what it would be best to do.

'I had a friend once called Maudsley, who went to the bad, and has just been serving his time in Pentonville. One day he had met me, and fell into talk about the ways of thieves, and how they could get rid of what they stole. I knew that he would be true to me, for I knew one or two things about him; so I made up my mind to go right on to Kilburn, where he lived, and take him into my confidence. He would show me how to turn the stone into money. But how to get to him in safety? I thought of the agonies I had gone through in coming from the hotel. I might at any moment be seized and searched, and there would be the stone in my waistcoat pocket. I was leaning against the wall at the time and looking at the geese which were waddling about round my feet, and suddenly an idea came into my head which showed me how I could beat the best detective that ever lived.

'My sister had told me some weeks before that I might have the pick of her geese for a Christmas present, and I knew that she was always as good as her word. I would take my goose now, and in it I would carry my stone to Kilburn. There was a little shed in the yard, and behind this I drove one of the birds – a fine big one, white, with a barred tail. I caught it, and prying its bill open, I thrust the stone down its throat as far as my finger could reach. The bird gave a gulp, and I felt the stone pass along its gullet and down into its crop. But the creature flapped and struggled, and out came my sister to know what was the matter. As I turned to speak to her the brute broke loose and fluttered off among the others.

'"Whatever were you doing with that bird, Jem?" says she.

'"Well," said I, "you said you'd give me one for Christmas, and I was feeling which was the fattest."

'"Oh," says she, "we've set yours aside for you – Jem's bird, we call it. It's the big white one over yonder. There's twenty-six of them, which makes one for you, and one for us, and two dozen for the market."

'"Thank you, Maggie," says I; "but if it is all the same to you, I'd rather have that one I was handling just now."

'"The other is a good three pound heavier," said she, "and we fattened it expressly for you."

'"Never mind. I'll have the other, and I'll take it now," said I.

'"Oh, just as you like," said she, a little huffed. "Which is it you want, then?"

'"That white one with the barred tail, right in the middle of the flock."

'"Oh, very well. Kill it and take it with you."

'Well, I did what she said, Mr Holmes, and I carried the bird all the way to Kilburn. I told my pal what I had done, for he was a man that it was easy to tell a thing like that to. He laughed until he choked, and we got a knife and opened the goose. My heart turned to water, for there was no sign of the stone, and I knew that some terrible mistake had occurred. I left the bird, rushed back to my sister's and hurried into the back yard. There was not a bird to be seen there.

'"Where are they all, Maggie?" I cried.

'"Gone to the dealer's, Jem."

'"Which dealer's?"

'"Breckinridge, of Covent Garden."

'"But was there another with a barred tail?" I asked, "the same as the one I chose?"

'"Yes, Jem; there were two barred-tailed ones, and I could never tell them apart."

'Well, then, of course I saw it all, and I ran off as hard as my feet would carry me to this man Breckinridge; but he had sold the lot at once, and not one word would he tell me as to where they had gone.

You heard him yourselves to-night. Well, he has always answered me like that. My sister thinks that I am going mad. Sometimes I think that I am myself. And now – and now I am myself a branded thief, without ever having touched the wealth for which I sold my character. God help me! God help me!' He burst into convulsive sobbing, with his face buried in his hands.

There was a long silence, broken only by his heavy breathing and by the measured tapping of Sherlock Holmes' finger-tips upon the edge of the table. Then my friend rose and threw open the door.

'Get out!' said he.

'What, sir! Oh, Heaven bless you!'

'No more words. Get out!'

And no more words were needed. There was a rush, a clatter upon the stairs, the bang of a door and the crisp rattle of running footfalls from the street.

'After all, Watson,' said Holmes, reaching up his hand for his clay pipe, 'I am not retained by the police to supply their deficiencies. If Horner were in danger it would be another thing; but this fellow will not appear against him, and the case must collapse. I suppose that I am commuting a felony, but it is just possible that I am saving a soul. This fellow will not go wrong again; he is too terribly frightened. Send him to gaol now, and you make him a gaol-bird for life. Besides, it is the season of forgiveness. Chance has put in our way a most singular and whimsical problem, and its solution is its own reward. If you will have the goodness to touch the bell, Doctor, we will begin another investigation, in which, also a bird will be the chief feature.'

THE PIPER AT THE GATES OF DAWN – AN EXCERPT FROM *THE WIND IN THE WILLOWS*

Kenneth Grahame

The Willow-Wren was twittering his thin little song, hidden himself in the dark selvedge of the river bank. Though it was past ten o'clock at night, the sky still clung to and retained some lingering skirts of light from the departed day; and the sullen heats of the torrid afternoon broke up and rolled away at the dispersing touch of the cool fingers of the short midsummer night. Mole lay stretched on the bank, still panting from the stress of the fierce day that had been cloudless from dawn to late sunset, and waited for his friend to return. He had been on the river with some companions, leaving the Water Rat free to keep an engagement of long standing with Otter; and he had come back to find the house dark and deserted, and no sign of Rat, who was doubtless keeping it up late with his old comrade. It was still too hot to think of staying indoors, so he lay on some cool dock-leaves, and thought over the past day and its doings, and how very good they all had been.

The Rat's light footfall was presently heard approaching over the parched grass. 'O, the blessed coolness!' he said, and sat down, gazing thoughtfully into the river, silent and pre-occupied.

'You stayed to supper, of course?' said the Mole presently.

'Simply had to,' said the Rat. 'They wouldn't hear of my going before. You know how kind they always are. And they made things as jolly for me as ever they could, right up to the moment I left. But I felt a brute all the time, as it was clear to me they were very unhappy, though they tried to hide it. Mole, I'm afraid they're in trouble. Little Portly is missing again; and you know what a lot his father thinks of him, though he never says much about it.'

'What, that child?' said the Mole lightly. 'Well, suppose he is; why worry about it? He's always straying off and getting lost, and turning up again; he's so adventurous. But no harm ever happens to him. Everybody hereabouts knows him and likes him, just as they do old Otter, and you may be sure some animal or other will come across him and bring him back again all right. Why, we've found him ourselves, miles from home, and quite self-possessed and cheerful!'

'Yes; but this time it's more serious,' said the Rat gravely. 'He's been missing for some days now, and the Otters have hunted everywhere, high and low, without finding the slightest trace. And they've asked every animal, too, for miles around, and no one knows anything about him. Otter's evidently more anxious than he'll admit. I got out of him that young Portly hasn't learnt to swim very well yet, and I can see he's thinking of the weir. There's a lot of water coming down still, considering the time of the year, and the place always had a fascination for the child. And then there are – well, traps and things – *you* know. Otter's not the fellow to be nervous about any son of his before it's time. And now he *is* nervous. When I left, he came out with me – said he wanted some air, and talked about stretching his legs. But I could see it wasn't that, so I drew him out and pumped him, and got it all from him at last. He was going to spend the night watching by the ford. You know the place where the old ford used to be, in by-gone days before they built the bridge?'

'I know it well,' said the Mole. 'But why should Otter choose to watch there?'

'Well, it seems that it was there he gave Portly his first swimming-lesson,' continued the Rat. 'From that shallow, gravelly spit near the bank. And it was there he used to teach him fishing, and there young Portly caught his first fish, of which he was so very proud. The child loved the spot, and Otter thinks that if he came wandering back from wherever he is – if he *is* anywhere by this time, poor little chap – he might make for the ford he was so fond of; or if he came across it he'd remember it well, and stop there and play, perhaps. So Otter goes there every night and watches – on the chance, you know, just on the chance!'

They were silent for a time, both thinking of the same thing – the lonely, heart-sore animal, crouched by the ford, watching and waiting, the long night through – on the chance.

'Well, well,' said the Rat presently, 'I suppose we ought to be thinking about turning in.' But he never offered to move.

'Rat,' said the Mole, 'I simply can't go and turn in, and go to sleep, and *do* nothing, even though there doesn't seem to be anything to be done. We'll get the boat out, and paddle up stream. The moon will be up in an hour or so, and then we will search as well as we can – anyhow, it will be better than going to bed and doing *nothing.*'

'Just what I was thinking myself,' said the Rat. 'It's not the sort of night for bed anyhow; and daybreak is not so very far off, and then we may pick up some news of him from early risers as we go along.'

They got the boat out, and the Rat took the sculls, paddling with caution. Out in midstream, there was a clear, narrow track that faintly reflected the sky; but wherever shadows fell on the water from bank, bush or tree, they were as solid to all appearance as the banks themselves, and the Mole had to steer with judgment accordingly. Dark and deserted as it was, the night was full of small noises, song and chatter and rustling, telling of the busy little population who were up and about, plying their trades and vocations through the night till sunshine should fall on them at last and send them off to their well-earned repose. The water's own noises, too, were more apparent than by day, its gurglings and 'cloops' more unexpected and near at hand; and constantly they started at what seemed a sudden clear call from an actual articulate voice.

The line of the horizon was clear and hard against the sky, and in one particular quarter it showed black against a silvery climbing phosphorescence that grew and grew. At last, over the rim of the waiting earth the moon lifted with slow majesty till it swung clear of the horizon and rode off, free of moorings; and once more they began to see surfaces – meadows wide-spread, and quiet gardens, and the river itself from bank to bank, all softly disclosed, all washed clean of mystery and terror, all radiant again as by day, but with a difference that was tremendous. Their old haunts greeted them again in other raiment, as if they had slipped away and put on this pure new apparel and come quietly back, smiling as they shyly waited to see if they would be recognized again under it.

Fastening their boat to a willow, the friends landed in this silent, silver kingdom, and patiently explored the hedges, the hollow trees, the runnels and their little culverts, the ditches and dry water-ways. Embarking again and crossing over, they worked their way up the stream in this manner, while the moon, serene and detached in a cloudless sky, did what she could, though so far off, to help them in their quest; till her hour came and she sank earthwards reluctantly, and left them, and mystery once more held field and river.

Then a change began slowly to declare itself. The horizon became clearer, field and tree came more into sight, and somehow with a different look; the mystery began to drop away from them. A bird piped suddenly, and was still; and a light breeze sprang up and set the reeds and bulrushes rustling. Rat, who was in the stern of the boat, while Mole sculled, sat up suddenly and listened with a passionate intentness. Mole, who with gentle strokes was just keeping the boat moving while he scanned the banks with care, looked at him with curiosity.

'It's gone!' sighed the Rat, sinking back in his seat again. 'So beautiful and strange and new. Since it was to end so soon, I almost wish I had never heard it. For it has roused a longing in me that is pain, and nothing seems worth while but just to hear that sound once more and go on listening to it for ever. No! There it is again!' he cried, alert once more. Entranced, he was silent for a long space, spellbound.

'Now it passes on and I begin to lose it,' he said presently. 'O Mole! the beauty of it! The merry bubble and joy, the thin, clear, happy call of the distant piping! Such music I never dreamed of, and the call in it is stronger even than the music is sweet! Row on, Mole, row! For the music and the call must be for us.'

The Mole, greatly wondering, obeyed. 'I hear nothing myself,' he said, 'but the wind playing in the reeds and rushes and osiers.'

The Rat never answered, if indeed he heard. Rapt, transported, trembling, he was possessed in all his senses by this new divine thing that caught up his helpless soul and swung and dandled it, a powerless but happy infant in a strong sustaining grasp.

In silence Mole rowed steadily, and soon they came to a point where the river divided, a long backwater branching off to one side. With a slight movement of his head Rat, who had long dropped the rudder-lines, directed the rower to take the backwater. The creeping tide of light gained and gained, and now they could see the colour of the flowers that gemmed the water's edge.

'Clearer and nearer still,' cried the Rat joyously. 'Now you must surely hear it! Ah – at last – I see you do!'

Breathless and transfixed the Mole stopped rowing as the liquid run of that glad piping broke on him like a wave, caught him up and possessed him utterly. He saw the tears on his comrade's cheeks, and bowed his head and understood. For a space they hung there, brushed by the purple loose-strife that fringed the bank; then the clear imperious summons that marched hand-in-hand with the intoxicating melody imposed its will on Mole, and mechanically he bent to his oars again. And the light grew steadily stronger, but no birds sang as they were wont to do at the approach of dawn; and but for the heavenly music all was marvellously still.

On either side of them, as they glided onwards, the rich meadow-grass seemed that morning of a freshness and a greenness unsurpassable. Never had they noticed the roses so vivid, the willow-herb so riotous, the meadow-sweet so odorous and pervading. Then the murmur of the approaching weir began to hold the air, and they felt a consciousness that they were nearing the end, whatever it might be, that surely awaited their expedition.

A wide half-circle of foam and glinting lights and shining shoulders of green water, the great weir closed the backwater from bank to bank, troubled all the quiet surface with twirling eddies and floating foam-streaks, and deadened all other sounds with its solemn and soothing rumble. In midmost of the stream, embraced in the weir's shimmering arm-spread, a small island lay anchored, fringed close with willow and silver birch and alder. Reserved, shy, but full of significance, it hid whatever it might hold behind a veil, keeping it till the hour should come, and, with the hour, those who were called and chosen.

Slowly, but with no doubt or hesitation whatever, and in something of a solemn expectancy, the two animals passed through the broken tumultuous water and moored their boat at the flowery margin of the island. In silence they landed, and pushed through the blossom and scented herbage and undergrowth that led up to the level ground, till they stood on a little lawn of a marvellous green, set round with Nature's own orchard-trees – crab-apple, wild cherry and sloe.

'This is the place of my song-dream, the place the music played to me,' whispered the Rat, as if in a trance. 'Here, in this holy place, here if anywhere, surely we shall find Him!'

Then suddenly the Mole felt a great Awe fall upon him, an awe that turned his muscles to water, bowed his head, and rooted his feet to the ground. It was no panic terror – indeed he felt wonderfully at peace and happy – but it was an awe that smote and held him and, without seeing, he knew it could only mean that some august Presence was very, very near. With difficulty he turned to look for his friend and saw him at his side cowed, stricken and trembling violently. And still there was utter silence in the populous bird-haunted branches around them; and still the light grew and grew.

Perhaps he would never have dared to raise his eyes, but that, though the piping was now hushed, the call and the summons seemed still dominant and imperious. He might not refuse, were Death himself waiting to strike him instantly, once he had looked with mortal eye on things rightly kept hidden. Trembling he obeyed, and raised his humble head; and then, in that utter clearness of the imminent dawn, while Nature, flushed with fullness of incredible colour, seemed to hold her breath for the event, he looked in the very eyes of the Friend and Helper; saw the backward sweep of the curved horns, gleaming in the growing daylight; saw the stern, hooked nose between the kindly eyes that were looking down on them humorously, while the bearded mouth broke into a half-smile at the corners; saw the rippling muscles on the arm that lay across the broad chest, the long supple hand still holding the pan-pipes only just fallen away from the parted lips; saw the splendid curves of the shaggy limbs disposed in majestic ease on the sward; saw, last of all, nestling between his very hooves, sleeping soundly in entire peace and contentment, the little, round, podgy, childish form of the baby otter. All this he saw, for one moment breathless and intense, vivid on the morning sky; and still, as he looked, he lived; and still, as he lived, he wondered.

'Rat!' he found breath to whisper, shaking. 'Are you afraid?'

'Afraid?' murmured the Rat, his eyes shining with unutterable love. 'Afraid! Of *Him*? O, never, never! And yet – and yet – O, Mole, I am afraid!'

Then the two animals, crouching to the earth, bowed their heads and did worship.

Sudden and magnificent, the sun's broad golden disc showed itself over the horizon facing them; and the first rays, shooting across the level water-meadows, took the animals full in the eyes and dazzled them. When they were able to look once more, the Vision had vanished, and the air was full of the carol of birds that hailed the dawn.

As they stared blankly in dumb misery deepening as they slowly realized all they had seen and all they had lost, a capricious little breeze, dancing up from the surface of the water, tossed the aspens, shook the dewy roses and blew lightly and caressingly in their faces; and with its soft touch came instant oblivion. For this is the last best gift that the kindly demi-god is careful to bestow on those to whom he has revealed himself in their helping: the gift of forgetfulness. Lest the awful remembrance should remain and grow, and overshadow mirth and pleasure, and the great haunting memory should spoil all the after-lives of little animals helped out of difficulties, in order that they should be happy and lighthearted as before.

Mole rubbed his eyes and stared at Rat, who was looking about him in a puzzled sort of way. 'I beg your pardon; what did you say, Rat?' he asked.

'I think I was only remarking,' said Rat slowly, 'that this was the right sort of place, and that here, if anywhere, we should find him. And look! Why, there he is, the little fellow!' And with a cry of delight he ran towards the slumbering Portly.

But Mole stood still a moment, held in thought. As one wakened suddenly from a beautiful dream, who struggles to recall it, and can re-capture nothing but a dim sense of the beauty of it, the beauty! Till that, too, fades away in its turn, and the dreamer bitterly accepts the hard, cold waking and all its penalties; so Mole, after struggling with his memory for a brief space, shook his head sadly and followed the Rat.

Portly woke up with a joyous squeak, and wriggled with pleasure at the sight of his father's friends, who had played with him so often in past days. In a moment, however, his face grew blank, and he fell to hunting round in a circle with pleading whine. As a child that has fallen happily asleep in its nurse's arms, and wakes to find itself alone and laid in a strange place, and searches corners and cupboards, and runs from room to room, despair growing silently in its heart, even so Portly searched the island and searched, dogged and unwearying, till at last the black moment came for giving it up, and sitting down and crying bitterly.

The Mole ran quickly to comfort the little animal; but Rat, lingering, looked long and doubtfully at certain hoof-marks deep in the sward.

'Some—great—animal—has been here,' he murmured slowly and thoughtfully; and stood musing, musing; his mind strangely stirred.

'Come along, Rat!' called the Mole. 'Think of poor Otter, waiting up there by the ford!'

Portly had soon been comforted by the promise of a treat – a jaunt on the river in Mr Rat's real boat; and the two animals conducted him to the water's side, placed him securely between them in the bottom of the boat, and paddled off down the backwater. The sun was fully up by now, and hot on them, birds sang lustily and without restraint, and flowers smiled and nodded from either bank, but somehow – so thought the animals – with less of richness and blaze of colour than they seemed to remember seeing quite recently somewhere – they wondered where.

The main river reached again, they turned the boat's head upstream, towards the point where they knew their friend was keeping his lonely vigil. As they drew near the familiar ford, the Mole took the boat in to the bank, and they lifted Portly out and set him on his legs on the tow-path, gave him his marching orders and a friendly farewell pat on the back, and shoved out into mid-stream. They watched the little animal as he waddled along the path contentedly and with importance; watched him till they saw his muzzle suddenly lift and his waddle break into a clumsy amble as he quickened his pace with shrill whines and wriggles of recognition. Looking up the river, they could see Otter start up, tense and rigid, from out of the shallows where he crouched in dumb patience, and could hear his amazed and joyous bark as he bounded up through the osiers on to the path. Then the Mole, with a strong pull on one oar, swung the boat round and let the full stream bear them down again whither it would, their quest now happily ended.

'I feel strangely tired, Rat,' said the Mole, leaning wearily over his oars as the boat drifted. 'It's being up all night, you'll say, perhaps; but that's nothing. We do as much half the nights of the week, at this time of the year. No; I feel as if I had been through something very exciting and rather terrible, and it was just over; and yet nothing particular has happened.'

'Or something very surprising and splendid and beautiful,' murmured the Rat, leaning back and closing his eyes. 'I feel just as you do, Mole; simply dead tired, though not body tired. It's lucky we've got the stream with us, to take us home. Isn't it jolly to feel the sun again, soaking into one's bones! And hark to the wind playing in the reeds!'

'It's like music – far away music,' said the Mole nodding drowsily.

'So I was thinking,' murmured the Rat, dreamful and languid. 'Dance-music – the lilting sort that runs on without a stop – but with words in it, too – it passes into words and out of them again – I catch them at intervals – then it is dance-music once more, and then nothing but the reeds' soft thin whispering.'

'You hear better than I,' said the Mole sadly. 'I cannot catch the words.'

'Let me try and give you them,' said the Rat softly, his eyes still closed. 'Now it is turning into words again – faint but clear – *Lest the awe should dwell – And turn your frolic to fret – You shall look on my power at the helping hour – But then you shall forget!* Now the reeds take it up – *forget, forget,* they sigh, and it dies away in a rustle and a whisper. Then the voice returns—

'*Lest limbs be reddened and rent – I spring the trap that is set – As I loose the snare you may glimpse me there – For surely you shall forget!* Row nearer, Mole, nearer to the reeds! It is hard to catch, and grows each minute fainter.

'*Helper and healer, I cheer – Small waifs in the woodland wet – Strays I find in it, wounds I bind in it – Bidding them all forget!* Nearer, Mole, nearer! No, it is no good; the song has died away into reed-talk.'

'But what do the words mean?' asked the wondering Mole.

'That I do not know,' said the Rat simply. 'I passed them on to you as they reached me. Ah! now they return again, and this time full and clear! This time, at last, it is the real, the unmistakable thing, simple – passionate – perfect—'

'Well, let's have it, then,' said the Mole, after he had waited patiently for a few minutes, half-dozing in the hot sun.

But no answer came. He looked, and understood the silence. With a smile of much happiness on his face, and something of a listening look still lingering there, the weary Rat was fast asleep.

BEAUTY AND THE BEAST

Madame de Villeneuve

Once upon a time, in a very far-off country, there lived a
merchant who had been so fortunate in all his undertakings
that he was enormously rich. As he had, however, six sons
and six daughters, he found that his money was not too much to
let them all have everything they fancied, as they were accustomed
to do.

But one day a most unexpected misfortune befell them. Their
house caught fire and was speedily burnt to the ground, with all the
splendid furniture, the books, pictures, gold, silver and precious
goods it contained; and this was only the beginning of their
troubles. Their father, who had until this moment prospered in all
ways, suddenly lost every ship he had upon the sea, either by dint of
pirates, shipwreck or fire. Then he heard that his clerks in distant
countries, whom he trusted entirely, had proved unfaithful; and at
last from great wealth he fell into the direst poverty.

All that he had left was a little house in a desolate place at least
a hundred leagues from the town in which he had lived, and to this
he was forced to retreat with his children, who were in despair at
the idea of leading such a different life. Indeed, the daughters at first
hoped that their friends, who had been so numerous while they
were rich, would insist on their staying in their houses now they no

longer possessed one. But they soon found that they were left alone, and that their former friends even attributed their misfortunes to their own extravagance, and showed no intention of offering them any help. So nothing was left for them but to take their departure to the cottage, which stood in the midst of a dark forest, and seemed to be the most dismal place upon the face of the earth. As they were too poor to have any servants, the girls had to work hard, like peasants, and the sons, for their part, cultivated the fields to earn their living. Roughly clothed, and living in the simplest way, the girls regretted unceasingly the luxuries and amusements of their former life; only the youngest tried to be brave and cheerful. She had been as sad as anyone when misfortune overtook her father, but, soon recovering her natural gaiety, she set to work to make the best of things, to amuse her father and brothers as well as she could, and to try to persuade her sisters to join her in dancing and singing. But they would do nothing of the sort, and, because she was not as doleful as themselves, they declared that this miserable life was all she was fit for. But she was really far prettier and cleverer than they were; indeed, she was so lovely that she was always called Beauty. After two years, when they were all beginning to get used to their new life, something happened to disturb their tranquillity. Their father received the news that one of his ships, which he had believed to be lost, had come safely into port with a rich cargo. All the sons and daughters at once thought that their poverty was at an end, and wanted to set out directly for the town; but their father, who was more prudent, begged them to wait a little, and, though it was harvest time, and he could ill be spared, determined to go himself first, to make inquiries. Only the youngest daughter had any doubt but that they would soon again be as rich as they were before, or at least rich enough to live comfortably in some town where they would find amusement and companions once more.

So they all loaded their father with commissions for jewels and dresses which it would have taken a fortune to buy; only Beauty, feeling sure that it was of no use, did not ask for anything. Her father, noticing her silence, said: 'And what shall I bring for you, Beauty?'

'The only thing I wish for is to see you come home safely,' she answered.

But this only vexed her sisters, who fancied she was blaming them for having asked for such costly things. Her father, however, was pleased, but as he thought that at her age she certainly ought to like pretty presents, he told her to choose something.

'Well, dear father,' she said, 'as you insist upon it, I beg that you will bring me a rose. I have not seen one since we came here, and I love them so much.'

So the merchant set out and reached the town as quickly as possible, but only to find that his former companions, believing him to be dead, had divided between them the goods which the ship had brought; and after six months of trouble and expense he found himself as poor as when he started, having been able to recover only just enough to pay the cost of his journey. To make matters worse, he was obliged to leave the town in the most terrible weather, so that by the time he was within a few leagues of his home he was almost exhausted with cold and fatigue. Though he knew it would take some hours to get through the forest, he was so anxious to be at his journey's end that he resolved to go on; but night overtook him, and the deep snow and bitter frost made it impossible for his horse to carry him any further. Not a house was to be seen; the only shelter he could get was the hollow trunk of a great tree, and there he crouched all the night which seemed to him the longest he had ever known. In spite of his weariness the howling of the wolves kept him awake, and even when at last the day broke he was not much better off, for the falling snow had covered up every path, and he did not know which way to turn.

At length he made out some sort of track, and though at the beginning it was so rough and slippery that he fell down more than once, it presently became easier, and led him into an avenue of trees which ended in a splendid castle. It seemed to the merchant very strange that no snow had fallen in the avenue, which was entirely composed of orange trees, covered with flowers and fruit. When he reached the first court of the castle he saw before him a flight of agate steps, and went up them, and passed through several splendidly furnished rooms. The pleasant warmth of the air revived him, and he felt very hungry; but there seemed to be nobody in all this vast and splendid palace whom he could ask to give him something to eat. Deep silence reigned everywhere, and at last, tired of roaming through empty rooms and galleries, he stopped in a room smaller than the rest, where a clear fire was burning and a couch was drawn up closely to it. Thinking that this must be prepared for someone who was expected, he sat down to wait till he should come, and very soon fell into a sweet sleep.

When his extreme hunger wakened him after several hours, he was still alone; but a little table, upon which was a good dinner, had been drawn up close to him, and, as he had eaten nothing for twenty-four hours, he lost no time in beginning his meal, hoping that he might soon have an opportunity of thanking his considerate entertainer, whoever it might be. But no one appeared, and even after another long sleep, from which he awoke completely refreshed, there was no sign of anybody, though a fresh meal of dainty cakes and fruit was prepared upon the little table at his elbow. Being naturally timid, the silence began to terrify him, and he resolved to search once more through all the rooms; but it was of no use. Not even a servant was to be seen; there was no sign of life in the palace! He began to wonder what he should do, and to amuse himself by pretending that all the treasures he saw were his own, and considering how he would divide them among his children. Then he went down into the garden, and though it was winter everywhere else, here the sun shone, and the birds sang, and the flowers bloomed, and the air was soft and sweet. The merchant, in ecstasies with all he saw and heard, said to himself:

'All this must be meant for me. I will go this minute and bring my children to share all these delights.'

In spite of being so cold and weary when he reached the castle, he had taken his horse to the stable and fed it. Now he thought he would saddle it for his homeward journey, and he turned down the path which led to the stable. This path had a hedge of roses on each side of it, and the merchant thought he had never seen or smelt such exquisite flowers. They reminded him of his promise to Beauty, and he stopped and had just gathered one to take to her when he was startled by a strange noise behind him. Turning round, he saw a frightful Beast, which seemed to be very angry and said, in a terrible voice:

'Who told you that you might gather my roses? Was it not enough that I allowed you to be in my palace and was kind to you? This is the way you show your gratitude, by stealing my flowers! But your insolence shall not go unpunished.' The merchant, terrified by these furious words, dropped the fatal rose, and, throwing himself on his knees, cried: 'Pardon me, noble sir. I am truly grateful to you for your hospitality, which was so magnificent that I could not imagine that you would be offended by my taking such a little thing as a rose.' But the Beast's anger was not lessened by this speech.

'You are very ready with excuses and flattery,' he cried; 'but that will not save you from the death you deserve.'

'Alas!' thought the merchant, 'if my daughter could only know what danger her rose has brought me into!'

And in despair he began to tell the Beast all his misfortunes, and the reason of his journey, not forgetting to mention Beauty's request.

'A king's ransom would hardly have procured all that my other daughters asked,' he said: 'but I thought that I might at least take Beauty her rose. I beg you to forgive me, for you see I meant no harm.'

The Beast considered for a moment, and then he said, in a less furious tone:

'I will forgive you on one condition – that is, that you will give me one of your daughters.'

'Ah!' cried the merchant, 'if I were cruel enough to buy my own life at the expense of one of my children's, what excuse could I invent to bring her here?'

'No excuse would be necessary,' answered the Beast. 'If she comes at all she must come willingly. On no other condition will I have her. See if any one of them is courageous enough, and loves you well enough to come and save your life. You seem to be an honest man, so I will trust you to go home. I give you a month to see if either of your daughters will come back with you and stay here, to let you go free. If neither of them is willing, you must come alone, after bidding them good-bye for ever, for then you will belong to me. And do not imagine that you can hide from me, for if you fail to keep your word I will come and fetch you!' added the Beast grimly.

The merchant accepted this proposal, though he did not really think any of his daughters could be persuaded to come. He promised to return at the time appointed, and then, anxious to escape from the presence of the Beast, he asked permission to set off at once. But the Beast answered that he could not go until next day.

'Then you will find a horse ready for you,' he said. 'Now go and eat your supper, and await my orders.'

The poor merchant, more dead than alive, went back to his room, where the most delicious supper was already served on the little table which was drawn up before a blazing fire. But he was too terrified to eat, and only tasted a few of the dishes, for fear the Beast should be angry if he did not obey his orders. When he had finished he heard a great noise in the next room, which he knew meant that the Beast was coming. As he could do nothing to escape his visit, the only thing that remained was to seem as little afraid as possible; so when the Beast appeared and asked roughly if he had supped well, the merchant answered humbly that he had, thanks to his host's kindness. Then the Beast warned him to remember their agreement, and to prepare his daughter exactly for what she had to expect.

'Do not get up to-morrow,' he added, 'until you see the sun and hear a golden bell ring. Then you will find your breakfast waiting for you here, and the horse you are to ride will be ready in the courtyard. He will also bring you back again when you come with your daughter a month hence. Farewell. Take a rose to Beauty, and remember your promise!'

The merchant was only too glad when the Beast went away, and though he could not sleep for sadness, he lay down until the sun rose. Then, after a hasty breakfast, he went to gather Beauty's rose, and mounted his horse, which carried him off so swiftly that in an instant he had lost sight of the palace, and he was still wrapped in gloomy thoughts when it stopped before the door of the cottage.

His sons and daughters, who had been very uneasy at his long absence, rushed to meet him, eager to know the result of his journey, which, seeing him mounted upon a splendid horse and wrapped in a rich mantle, they supposed to be favourable. He hid the truth from them at first, only saying sadly to Beauty as he gave her the rose:

'Here is what you asked me to bring you; you little know what it has cost.'

But this excited their curiosity so greatly that presently he told them his adventures from beginning to end, and then they were all very unhappy. The girls lamented loudly over their lost hopes, and the sons declared that their father should not return to this terrible castle, and began to make plans for killing the Beast if it should come to fetch him. But he reminded them that he had promised to go back. Then the girls were very angry with Beauty, and said it was all her fault, and that if she had asked for something sensible this would never have happened, and complained bitterly that they should have to suffer for her folly.

Poor Beauty, much distressed, said to them:

'I have, indeed, caused this misfortune, but I assure you I did it innocently. Who could have guessed that to ask for a rose in the middle of summer would cause so much misery? But as I did the mischief it is only just that I should suffer for it. I will therefore go back with my father to keep his promise.'

At first nobody would hear of this arrangement, and her father and brothers, who loved her dearly, declared that nothing should make them let her go; but Beauty was firm. As the time drew near she divided all her little possessions between her sisters, and said good-bye to everything she loved, and when the fatal day came she encouraged and cheered her father as they mounted together the horse which had brought him back. It seemed to fly rather than gallop, but so smoothly that Beauty was not frightened; indeed, she would have enjoyed the journey if she had not feared what might happen to her at the end of it. Her father still tried to persuade her to go back, but in vain. While they were talking the night fell, and then, to their great surprise, wonderful coloured lights began to shine in all directions, and splendid fireworks blazed out before them; all the forest was illuminated by them, and even felt pleasantly warm, though it had been bitterly cold before. This lasted until they reached the avenue of orange trees, where there were statues holding flaming torches, and when they got nearer to the palace they saw that it was illuminated from the roof to the ground, and music sounded softly from the courtyard. 'The Beast must be very hungry,' said Beauty, trying to laugh, 'if he makes all this rejoicing over the arrival of his prey.'

But, in spite of her anxiety, she could not help admiring all the wonderful things she saw.

The horse stopped at the foot of the flight of steps leading to the terrace, and when they had dismounted her father led her to the little room he had been in before, where they found a splendid fire burning, and the table daintily spread with a delicious supper.

The merchant knew that this was meant for them, and Beauty, who was rather less frightened now that she had passed through so many rooms and seen nothing of the Beast, was quite willing to begin, for her long ride had made her very hungry. But they had hardly finished their meal when the noise of the Beast's footsteps was heard approaching, and Beauty clung to her father in terror, which became all the greater when she saw how frightened he was. But when the Beast really appeared, though she trembled at the sight of him, she made a great effort to hide her terror, and saluted him respectfully.

This evidently pleased the Beast. After looking at her he said, in a tone that might have struck terror into the boldest heart, though he did not seem to be angry:

'Good-evening, old man. Good-evening, Beauty.'

The merchant was too terrified to reply, but Beauty answered sweetly: 'Good-evening, Beast.'

'Have you come willingly?' asked the Beast. 'Will you be content to stay here when your father goes away?'

Beauty answered bravely that she was quite prepared to stay.

'I am pleased with you,' said the Beast. 'As you have come of your own accord, you may stay. As for you, old man,' he added, turning to the merchant, 'at sunrise to-morrow you will take your departure. When the bell rings get up quickly and eat your breakfast, and you will find the same horse waiting to take you home; but remember that you must never expect to see my palace again.'

Then turning to Beauty, he said:

'Take your father into the next room, and help him to choose everything you think your brothers and sisters would like to have. You will find two travelling-trunks there; fill them as full as you can. It is only just that you should send them something very precious as a remembrance of yourself.'

Then he went away, after saying, 'Good-bye, Beauty; good-bye, old man'; and though Beauty was beginning to think with great dismay of her father's departure, she was afraid to disobey the Beast's orders; and they went into the next room, which had shelves and cupboards all round it. They were greatly surprised at the riches it contained. There were splendid dresses fit for a queen, with all the ornaments that were to be worn with them; and when Beauty opened the cupboards she was quite dazzled by the gorgeous jewels that lay in heaps upon every shelf. After choosing a vast quantity, which she divided between her sisters – for she had made a heap of the wonderful dresses for each of them – she opened the last chest, which was full of gold.

'I think, father,' she said, 'that, as the gold will be more useful to you, we had better take out the other things again, and fill the trunks with it.' So they did this; but the more they put in the more room there seemed to be, and at last they put back all the jewels and dresses they had taken out, and Beauty even added as many more of the jewels as she could carry at once; and then the trunks were not too full, but they were so heavy that an elephant could not have carried them!

'The Beast was mocking us,' cried the merchant; 'he must have pretended to give us all these things, knowing that I could not carry them away.'

'Let us wait and see,' answered Beauty. 'I cannot believe that he meant to deceive us. All we can do is to fasten them up and leave them ready.'

So they did this and returned to the little room, where, to their astonishment, they found breakfast ready. The merchant ate his with a good appetite, as the Beast's generosity made him believe that he might perhaps venture to come back soon and see Beauty. But she felt sure that her father was leaving her for ever, so she was very sad when the bell rang sharply for the second time, and warned them that the time had come for them to part. They went down into the courtyard, where two horses were waiting, one loaded with the two trunks, the other for him to ride. They were pawing the ground in their impatience to start, and the merchant was forced to bid Beauty a hasty farewell; and as soon as he was mounted he went off at such a pace that she lost sight of him in an instant. Then Beauty began to cry, and wandered sadly back to her own room. But she soon found that she was very sleepy, and as she had nothing better to do she lay down and instantly fell asleep. And then she dreamed that she was walking by a brook bordered with trees, and lamenting her sad fate, when a young prince, handsomer than anyone she had ever seen, and with a voice that went straight to her heart, came and said to her, 'Ah, Beauty! you are not so unfortunate as you suppose. Here you will be rewarded for all you have suffered elsewhere. Your every wish shall be gratified. Only try to find me out, no matter how I may be disguised, as I love you dearly, and in making me happy you will find your own happiness.

Be as true-hearted as you are beautiful, and we shall have nothing left to wish for.'

'What can I do, Prince, to make you happy?' said Beauty.

'Only be grateful,' he answered, 'and do not trust too much to your eyes. And, above all, do not desert me until you have saved me from my cruel misery.'

After this she thought she found herself in a room with a stately and beautiful lady, who said to her:

'Dear Beauty, try not to regret all you have left behind you, for you are destined to a better fate. Only do not let yourself be deceived by appearances.'

Beauty found her dreams so interesting that she was in no hurry to awake, but presently the clock roused her by calling her name softly twelve times, and then she got up and found her dressing-table set out with everything she could possibly want; and when her toilet was finished she found dinner was waiting in the room next to hers. But dinner does not take very long when you are all by yourself, and very soon she sat down cosily in the corner of a sofa, and began to think about the charming Prince she had seen in her dream.

'He said I could make him happy,' said Beauty to herself.

'It seems, then, that this horrible Beast keeps him a prisoner. How can I set him free? I wonder why they both told me not to trust to appearances? I don't understand it. But, after all, it was only a dream, so why should I trouble myself about it? I had better go and find something to do to amuse myself.'

So she got up and began to explore some of the many rooms of the palace.

The first she entered was lined with mirrors, and Beauty saw herself reflected on every side, and thought she had never seen such a charming room. Then a bracelet which was hanging from a chandelier caught her eye, and on taking it down she was greatly surprised to find that it held a portrait of her unknown admirer, just as she had seen him in her dream. With great delight she slipped the bracelet on her arm, and went on into a gallery of pictures, where she soon found a portrait of the same handsome Prince, as large as life, and so well painted that as she studied it he seemed to smile kindly at her. Tearing herself away from the portrait at last, she passed through into a room which contained every musical instrument under the sun, and here she amused herself for a long while in trying some of them, and singing until she was tired. The next room was a library, and she saw everything she had ever wanted to read, as well as everything she had read, and it seemed to her that a whole lifetime would not be enough to even read the names of the books, there were so many. By this time it was growing dusk, and wax candles in diamond and ruby candlesticks were beginning to light themselves in every room.

Beauty found her supper served just at the time she preferred to have it, but she did not see anyone or hear a sound, and, though her father had warned her that she would be alone, she began to find it rather dull.

But presently she heard the Beast coming, and wondered tremblingly if he meant to eat her up now.

However, as he did not seem at all ferocious, and only said gruffly:

'Good-evening, Beauty,' she answered cheerfully and managed to conceal her terror. Then the Beast asked her how she had been amusing herself, and she told him all the rooms she had seen.

Then he asked if she thought she could be happy in his palace; and Beauty answered that everything was so beautiful that she would be very hard to please if she could not be happy. And after about an hour's talk Beauty began to think that the Beast was not nearly so terrible as she had supposed at first. Then he got up to leave her, and said in his gruff voice:

'Do you love me, Beauty? Will you marry me?'

'Oh! what shall I say?' cried Beauty, for she was afraid to make the Beast angry by refusing.

'Say "yes" or "no" without fear,' he replied.

'Oh! no, Beast,' said Beauty hastily.

'Since you will not, good-night, Beauty,' he said.

And she answered, 'Good-night, Beast,' very glad to find that her refusal had not provoked him. And after he was gone she was very soon in bed and asleep, and dreaming of her unknown Prince. She thought he came and said to her:

'Ah, Beauty! why are you so unkind to me? I fear I am fated to be unhappy for many a long day still.'

And then her dreams changed, but the charming Prince figured in them all; and when morning came her first thought was to look at the portrait, and see if it was really like him, and she found that it certainly was.

This morning she decided to amuse herself in the garden, for the sun shone, and all the fountains were playing; but she was astonished to find that every place was familiar to her, and presently she came to the brook where the myrtle trees were growing where she had first met the Prince in her dream, and that made her think more than ever that he must be kept a prisoner by the Beast. When she was tired she went back to the palace, and found a new room full of materials for every kind of work – ribbons to make into bows, and silks to work into flowers. Then there was an aviary full of rare birds, which were so tame that they flew to Beauty as soon as they saw her, and perched upon her shoulders and her head.

'Pretty little creatures,' she said, 'how I wish that your cage was nearer to my room, that I might often hear you sing!'

So saying she opened a door, and found, to her delight, that it led into her own room, though she had thought it was quite the other side of the palace.

There were more birds in a room farther on, parrots and cockatoos that could talk, and they greeted Beauty by name; indeed, she found them so entertaining that she took one or two back to her room, and they talked to her while she was at supper; after which the Beast paid her his usual visit, and asked her the same questions as before, and then with a gruff 'good-night' he took his departure, and Beauty went to bed to dream of her mysterious Prince. The days passed swiftly in different amusements, and after a while Beauty found out another strange thing in the palace, which often pleased her when she was tired of being alone. There was one room which she had not noticed particularly; it was empty, except that under each of the windows stood a very comfortable chair; and the first time she had looked out of the window it had seemed to her that a black curtain prevented her from seeing anything outside. But the second time she went into the room, happening to be tired, she sat down in one of the chairs, when instantly the curtain was rolled aside, and a most amusing pantomime was acted before her; there were dances, and coloured lights, and music, and pretty dresses, and it was all so gay that Beauty was in ecstasies. After that she tried the other seven windows in turn, and there was some new and surprising entertainment to be seen from each of them, so that Beauty never could feel lonely any more. Every evening after supper the Beast came to see her, and always before saying good-night asked her in his terrible voice:

'Beauty, will you marry me?'

And it seemed to Beauty, now she understood him better, that when she said, 'No, Beast,' he went away quite sad. But her happy dreams of the handsome young Prince soon made her forget the poor Beast, and the only thing that at all disturbed her was to be constantly told to distrust appearances, to let her heart guide her, and not her eyes, and many other equally perplexing things, which, consider as she would, she could not understand.

So everything went on for a long time, until at last, happy as she was, Beauty began to long for the sight of her father and her brothers and sisters; and one night, seeing her look very sad, the Beast asked her what was the matter. Beauty had quite ceased to be afraid of him. Now she knew that he was really gentle in spite of his ferocious looks and his dreadful voice. So she answered that she was longing to see her home once more. Upon hearing this the Beast seemed sadly distressed, and cried miserably.

'Ah! Beauty, have you the heart to desert an unhappy Beast like this? What more do you want to make you happy? Is it because you hate me that you want to escape?'

'No, dear Beast,' answered Beauty softly, 'I do not hate you, and I should be very sorry never to see you any more, but I long to see my father again. Only let me go for two months, and I promise to come back to you and stay for the rest of my life.'

The Beast, who had been sighing dolefully while she spoke, now replied:

'I cannot refuse you anything you ask, even though it should cost me my life. Take the four boxes you will find in the room next to your own, and fill them with everything you wish to take with you. But remember your promise and come back when the two months are over, or you may have cause to repent it, for if you do not come in good time you will find your faithful Beast dead. You will not need any chariot to bring you back. Only say good-bye to all your brothers and sisters the night before you come away, and when you have gone to bed turn this ring round upon your finger and say firmly: "I wish to go back to my palace and see my Beast again."

Good-night, Beauty. Fear nothing, sleep peacefully, and before long you shall see your father once more.'

As soon as Beauty was alone she hastened to fill the boxes with all the rare and precious things she saw about her, and only when she was tired of heaping things into them did they seem to be full.

Then she went to bed, but could hardly sleep for joy. And when at last she did begin to dream of her beloved Prince she was grieved to see him stretched upon a grassy bank, sad and weary, and hardly like himself.

'What is the matter?' she cried.

He looked at her reproachfully, and said:

'How can you ask me, cruel one? Are you not leaving me to my death perhaps?'

'Ah! don't be so sorrowful,' cried Beauty; 'I am only going to assure my father that I am safe and happy. I have promised the Beast faithfully that I will come back, and he would die of grief if I did not keep my word!'

'What would that matter to you?' said the Prince 'Surely you would not care?'

'Indeed, I should be ungrateful if I did not care for such a kind Beast,' cried Beauty indignantly. 'I would die to save him from pain. I assure you it is not his fault that he is so ugly.'

Just then a strange sound woke her – someone was speaking not very far away; and opening her eyes she found herself in a room she had never seen before, which was certainly not nearly so splendid as those she was used to in the Beast's palace. Where could she be? She got up and dressed hastily, and then saw that the boxes she had packed the night before were all in the room. While she was wondering by what magic the Beast had transported them and herself to this strange place she suddenly heard her father's voice, and rushed out and greeted him joyfully. Her brothers and sisters were all astonished at her appearance, as they had never expected to see her again, and there was no end to the questions they asked her. She had also much to hear about what had happened to them while she was away, and of her father's journey home. But when they heard that she had only come to be with them for a short time, and then must go back to the Beast's palace for ever, they lamented loudly. Then Beauty asked her father what he thought could be the meaning of her strange dreams, and why the Prince constantly begged her not to trust to appearances. After much consideration, he answered: 'You tell me yourself that the Beast, frightful as he is, loves you dearly, and deserves your love and gratitude for his gentleness and kindness; I think the Prince must mean you to understand that you ought to reward him by doing as he wishes you to, in spite of his ugliness.'

Beauty could not help seeing that this seemed very probable; still, when she thought of her dear Prince who was so handsome, she did not feel at all inclined to marry the Beast. At any rate, for two months she need not decide, but could enjoy herself with her sisters. But though they were rich now, and lived in town again, and had plenty of acquaintances, Beauty found that nothing amused her very much; and she often thought of the palace, where she was so happy, especially as at home she never once dreamed of her dear Prince, and she felt quite sad without him.

Then her sisters seemed to have got quite used to being without her, and even found her rather in the way, so she would not have been sorry when the two months were over but for her father and brothers, who begged her to stay, and seemed so grieved at the thought of her departure that she had not the courage to say good-bye to them. Every day when she got up she meant to say it at night, and when night came she put it off again, until at last she had a dismal dream which helped her to make up her mind. She thought she was wandering in a lonely path in the palace gardens, when she heard groans which seemed to come from some bushes hiding the entrance of a cave, and running quickly to see what could be the matter, she found the Beast stretched out upon his side, apparently dying. He reproached her faintly with being the cause of his distress, and at the same moment a stately lady appeared, and said very gravely:

'Ah! Beauty, you are only just in time to save his life. See what happens when people do not keep their promises! If you had delayed one day more, you would have found him dead.'

Beauty was so terrified by this dream that the next morning she announced her intention of going back at once, and that very night she said good-bye to her father and all her brothers and sisters, and as soon as she was in bed she turned her ring round upon her finger, and said firmly, 'I wish to go back to my palace and see my Beast again,' as she had been told to do.

Then she fell asleep instantly, and only woke up to hear the clock saying 'Beauty, Beauty' twelve times in its musical voice, which told her at once that she was really in the palace once more. Everything was just as before, and her birds were so glad to see her! But Beauty thought she had never known such a long day, for she was so anxious to see the Beast again that she felt as if suppertime would never come.

But when it did come and no Beast appeared she was really frightened; so, after listening and waiting for a long time, she ran down into the garden to search for him. Up and down the paths and avenues ran poor Beauty, calling him in vain, for no one answered, and not a trace of him could she find; until at last, quite tired, she stopped for a minute's rest, and saw that she was standing opposite the shady path she had seen in her dream. She rushed down it, and, sure enough, there was the cave, and in it lay the

Beast – asleep, as Beauty thought. Quite glad to have found him, she ran up and stroked his head, but, to her horror, he did not move or open his eyes.

'Oh! he is dead; and it is all my fault,' said Beauty, crying bitterly.

But then, looking at him again, she fancied he still breathed, and, hastily fetching some water from the nearest fountain, she sprinkled it over his face, and, to her great delight, he began to revive.

'Oh! Beast, how you frightened me!' she cried. 'I never knew how much I loved you until just now, when I feared I was too late to save your life.'

'Can you really love such an ugly creature as I am?' said the Beast faintly. 'Ah! Beauty, you only came just in time. I was dying because I thought you had forgotten your promise. But go back now and rest, I shall see you again by and by.'

Beauty, who had half expected that he would be angry with her, was reassured by his gentle voice, and went back to the palace, where supper was awaiting her; and afterward the Beast came in as usual, and talked about the time she had spent with her father, asking if she had enjoyed herself, and if they had all been very glad to see her.

Beauty answered politely, and quite enjoyed telling him all that had happened to her. And when at last the time came for him to go, and he asked, as he had so often asked before, 'Beauty, will you marry me?'

She answered softly, 'Yes, dear Beast.'

As she spoke a blaze of light sprang up before the windows of the palace; fireworks crackled and guns banged, and across the avenue of orange trees, in letters all made of fire-flies, was written: 'Long live the Prince and his Bride.'

Turning to ask the Beast what it could all mean, Beauty found that he had disappeared, and in his place stood her long-loved Prince! At the same moment the wheels of a chariot were heard upon the terrace, and two ladies entered the room. One of them Beauty recognized as the stately lady she had seen in her dreams; the other was also so grand and queenly that Beauty hardly knew which to greet first.

But the one she already knew said to her companion:

'Well, Queen, this is Beauty, who has had the courage to rescue your son from the terrible enchantment. They love one another, and only your consent to their marriage is wanting to make them perfectly happy.'

'I consent with all my heart,' cried the Queen. 'How can I ever thank you enough, charming girl, for having restored my dear son to his natural form?'

And then she tenderly embraced Beauty and the Prince, who had meanwhile been greeting the Fairy and receiving her congratulations.

'Now,' said the Fairy to Beauty, 'I suppose you would like me to send for all your brothers and sisters to dance at your wedding?'

And so she did, and the marriage was celebrated the very next day with the utmost splendour, and Beauty and the Prince lived happily ever after.

MADAME IMBERT'S SAFE

Maurice Leblanc

At three o'clock in the morning, there were still half a dozen carriages in front of one of those small houses which form only the side of the boulevard Berthier. The door of that house opened, and a number of guests, male and female, emerged. The majority of them entered their carriages and were quickly driven away, leaving behind only two men who walked down Courcelles, where they parted, as one of them lived in that street. The other decided to return on foot as far as the Porte-Maillot. It was a beautiful winter's night, clear and cold; a night on which a brisk walk is agreeable and refreshing.

But, at the end of a few minutes, he had the disagreeable impression that he was being followed. Turning around, he saw a man skulking amongst the trees. He was not a coward; yet he felt it advisable to increase his speed. Then his pursuer commenced to run; and he deemed it prudent to draw his revolver and face him. But he had no time. The man rushed at him and attacked him violently. Immediately, they were engaged in a desperate struggle, wherein he felt that his unknown assailant had the advantage. He called for help, struggled and was thrown down on a pile of gravel, seized by the throat and gagged with a handkerchief that his assailant forced into his mouth. His eyes closed, and the man who was smothering him with his weight arose to defend himself against an unexpected attack. A blow from a cane and a kick from a boot; the man uttered two cries of pain, and fled, limping and cursing. Without deigning to pursue the fugitive, the new arrival stooped over the prostrate man and inquired:

'Are you hurt, monsieur?'

He was not injured, but he was dazed and unable to stand. His rescuer procured a carriage, placed him in it, and accompanied him to his house on the avenue de la Grande-Armée. On his arrival there, quite recovered, he overwhelmed his saviour with thanks.

'I owe you my life, monsieur, and I shall not forget it. I do not wish to alarm my wife at this time of night, but, to-morrow, she will be pleased to thank you personally. Come and breakfast with us. My name is Ludovic Imbert. May I ask yours?'

'Certainly, monsieur.'

And he handed Mon. Imbert a card bearing the name: 'Arsène Lupin'.

At that time, Arsène Lupin did not enjoy the celebrity which the Cahorn affair, his escape from the Prison de la Santé, and other brilliant exploits, afterwards gained for him. He had not even used the name of Arsène Lupin. The name was specially invented to designate the rescuer of Mon. Imbert; that is to say, it was in that affair that Arsène Lupin was baptized. Fully armed and ready for the fray, it is true, but lacking the resources and authority which command success, Arsène Lupin was then merely an apprentice in a profession wherein he soon became a master.

With what a thrill of joy he recalled the invitation he received that night! At last, he had reached his goal! At last, he had undertaken a task worthy of his strength and skill! The Imbert millions! What a magnificent feast for an appetite like his!

He prepared a special toilet for the occasion; a shabby frock-coat, baggy trousers, a frayed silk hat, well-worn collar and cuffs, all quite correct in form, but bearing the unmistakable stamp of poverty. His cravat was a black ribbon pinned with a false diamond. Thus accoutred, he descended the stairs of the house in which he lived at Montmartre. At the third floor, without stopping, he rapped on a closed door with the head of his cane. He walked to the exterior boulevards. A tram-car was passing. He boarded it, and someone who had been following him took a seat beside him. It was the lodger who occupied the room on the third floor. A moment later, this man said to Lupin:

'Well, governor?'

'Well, it is all fixed.'

'How?'

'I am going there to breakfast.'

'You breakfast – there!'

'Certainly. Why not? I rescued Mon. Ludovic Imbert from certain death at your hands. Mon. Imbert is not devoid of gratitude. He invited me to breakfast.'

There was a brief silence. Then the other said:

'But you are not going to throw up the scheme?'

'My dear boy,' said Lupin, 'when I arranged that little case of assault and battery, when I took the trouble at three o'clock in the morning, to rap you with my cane and tap you with my boot at the risk of injuring my only friend, it was not my intention to forego the advantages to be gained from a rescue so well arranged and executed. Oh! no, not at all.'

'But the strange rumours we hear about their fortune?'

'Never mind about that. For six months, I have worked on

this affair, investigated it, studied it, questioned the servants, the money-lenders and men of straw; for six months, I have shadowed the husband and wife. Consequently, I know what I am talking about. Whether the fortune came to them from old Brawford, as they pretend, or from some other source, I do not care. I know that it is a reality; that it exists. And some day it will be mine.'

'Bigre! One hundred millions!'

'Let us say ten, or even five – that is enough! They have a safe full of bonds, and there will be the devil to pay if I can't get my hands on them.'

The tram-car stopped at the Place de l'Etoile. The man whispered to Lupin:

'What am I to do now?'

'Nothing, at present. You will hear from me. There is no hurry.'

Five minutes later, Arsène Lupin was ascending the magnificent flight of stairs in the Imbert mansion, and Mon. Imbert introduced him to his wife. Madame Gervaise Imbert was a short plump woman, and very talkative. She gave Lupin a cordial welcome.

'I desired that we should be alone to entertain our saviour,' she said.

From the outset, they treated 'our saviour' as an old and valued friend. By the time dessert was served, their friendship was well cemented, and private confidences were being exchanged. Arsène related the story of his life, the life of his father as a magistrate, the sorrows of his childhood and his present difficulties. Gervaise, in turn, spoke of her youth, her marriage, the kindness of the aged Brawford, the hundred millions that she had inherited, the obstacles that prevented her from obtaining the enjoyment of her inheritance, the moneys she had been obliged to borrow at an exorbitant rate of interest, her endless contentions with Brawford's nephews and the litigation! the injunctions! in fact, everything!

'Just think of it, Monsieur Lupin, the bonds are there, in my husband's office, and if we detach a single coupon, we lose everything! They are there, in our safe, and we dare not touch them.'

Monsieur Lupin shivered at the bare idea of his proximity to so much wealth. Yet he felt quite certain that Monsieur Lupin would never suffer from the same difficulty as his fair hostess who declared she dare not touch the money.

'Ah! they are there!' he repeated, to himself; 'they are there!'

A friendship formed under such circumstances soon led to closer relations. When discreetly questioned, Arsène Lupin confessed his poverty and distress. Immediately, the unfortunate young man was appointed private secretary to the Imberts, husband and wife, at a salary of one hundred francs a month. He was to come to the house every day and receive orders for his work, and a room on the second floor was set apart as his office. This room was directly over Mon. Imbert's office.

Arsène soon realized that his position as secretary was essentially a sinecure. During the first two months, he had only four important letters to recopy, and was called only once to Mon. Imbert's office; consequently, he had only one opportunity to contemplate, officially, the Imbert safe. Moreover, he noticed that the secretary was not invited to the social functions of the employer. But he did not complain, as he preferred to remain, modestly, in the shade and maintain his peace and freedom.

However, he was not wasting any time. From the beginning, he made clandestine visits to Mon. Imbert's office, and paid his respects to the safe, which was hermetically closed. It was an immense block of iron and steel, cold and stern in appearance, which could not be forced open by the ordinary tools of the burglar's trade. But Arsène Lupin was not discouraged.

'Where force fails, cunning prevails,' he said to himself. 'The essential thing is to be on the spot when the opportunity occurs. In the meantime, I must watch and wait.'

He made immediately some preliminary preparations. After careful soundings made upon the floor of his room, he introduced a lead pipe which penetrated the ceiling of Mon. Imbert's office at a point between the two screeds of the cornice. By means of this pipe, he hoped to see and hear what transpired in the room below.

Henceforth, he passed his days stretched at full length upon the floor. He frequently saw the Imberts holding a consultation in front of the safe, investigating books and papers. When they turned the combination lock, he tried to learn the figures and the number of turns they made to the right and left. He watched their movements; he sought to catch their words. There was also a key necessary to complete the opening of the safe. What did they do with it? Did they hide it?

One day, he saw them leave the room without locking the safe. He descended the stairs quickly, and boldly entered the room. But they had returned.

'Oh! excuse me,' he said, 'I made a mistake in the door.'

'Come in, Monsieur Lupin, come in,' cried Madame Imbert, 'are you not at home here? We want your advice. What bonds should we sell? The foreign securities or the government annuities?'

'But the injunction?' said Lupin, with surprise.

'Oh! it doesn't cover all the bonds.'

She opened the door of the safe and withdrew a package of bonds. But her husband protested.

'No, no, Gervaise, it would be foolish to sell the foreign bonds. They are going up, whilst the annuities are as high as they ever will be. What do you think, my dear friend?'

The dear friend had no opinion; yet he advised the sacrifice of the annuities. Then she withdrew another package and, from it, she took a paper at random. It proved to be a three-per-cent annuity worth two thousand francs. Ludovic placed the package of bonds in his pocket. That afternoon, accompanied by his secretary, he sold the annuities to a stock-broker and realized forty-six thousand francs.

Whatever Madame Imbert might have said about it, Arsène Lupin did not feel at home in the Imbert house. On the contrary, his position there was a peculiar one. He learned that the servants did not even know his name. They called him 'monsieur'. Ludovic always spoke of him in the same way: 'You will tell monsieur. Has monsieur arrived?' Why that mysterious appellation?

Moreover, after their first outburst of enthusiasm, the Imberts seldom spoke to him, and, although treating him with the consideration due to a benefactor, they gave him little or no attention. They appeared to regard him as an eccentric character who did not like to be disturbed, and they respected his isolation as if it were a stringent rule on his part. On one occasion, while passing through the vestibule, he heard Madame Imbert say to the two gentlemen:

'He is such a barbarian!'

'Very well,' he said to himself, 'I am a barbarian.'

And, without seeking to solve the question of their strange conduct, he proceeded with the execution of his own plans. He had decided that he could not depend on chance, nor on the negligence of Madame Imbert, who carried the key of the safe, and who, on locking the safe, invariably scattered the letters forming the combination of the lock. Consequently, he must act for himself.

Finally, an incident precipitated matters; it was the vehement campaign instituted against the Imberts by certain newspapers that accused the Imberts of swindling. Arsène Lupin was present at certain family conferences when this new vicissitude was discussed. He decided that if he waited much longer, he would lose everything. During the next five days, instead of leaving the house about six o'clock, according to his usual habit, he locked himself in his room. It was supposed that he had gone out. But he was lying on the floor surveying the office of Mon. Imbert. During those five evenings, the favourable opportunity that he awaited did not take place. He left the house about midnight by a side door to which he held the key.

But on the sixth day, he learned that the Imberts, actuated by the malevolent insinuations of their enemies, proposed to make an inventory of the contents of the safe.

'They will do it to-night,' thought Lupin.

And truly, after dinner, Imbert and his wife retired to the office and commenced to examine the books of account and the securities contained in the safe. Thus, one hour after another passed away. He heard the servants go upstairs to their rooms. No one now remained on the first floor. Midnight! The Imberts were still at work.

'I must get to work,' murmured Lupin.

He opened his window. It opened on a court. Outside, everything was dark and quiet. He took from his desk a knotted rope, fastened it to the balcony in front of his window and quietly descended as far as the window below, which was that of Imbert's office. He stood upon the balcony for a moment, motionless, with attentive ear and watchful eye, but the heavy curtains effectually concealed the interior of the room. He cautiously pushed on the double window. If no one had examined it, it ought to yield to the slightest pressure, for, during the afternoon, he had so fixed the bolt that it would not enter the staple.

The window yielded to his touch. Then, with infinite care, he pushed it open sufficiently to admit his head. He parted the curtains a few inches, looked in and saw Mon. Imbert and his wife sitting in front of the safe, deeply absorbed in their work and speaking softly to each other at rare intervals.

He calculated the distance between him and them, considered the exact movements he would require to make in order to overcome them, one after the other, before they could call for help, and he was about to rush upon them, when Madame Imbert said:

'Ah! the room is getting quite cold. I am going to bed. And you, my dear?'

'I shall stay and finish.'

'Finish! Why, that will take you all night.'

'Not at all. An hour, at the most.'

She retired. Twenty minutes, thirty minutes passed. Arsène pushed the window a little farther open. The curtains shook. He pushed once more. Mon. Imbert turned, and, seeing the curtains blown by the wind, he rose to close the window.

There was not a cry, not the trace of struggle. With a few precise moments, and without causing him the least injury, Arsène stunned him, wrapped the curtain about his head, bound him hand and foot, and did it all in such a manner that Mon. Imbert had no opportunity to recognize his assailant.

Quickly, he approached the safe, seized two packages that he placed under his arm, left the office and opened the servants' gate. A carriage was stationed in the street.

'Take that, first – and follow me,' he said to the coachman. He returned to the office, and, in two trips, they emptied the safe. Then Arsène went to his own room, removed the rope, and all other traces of his clandestine work.

A few hours later, Arsène Lupin and his assistant examined the stolen goods. Lupin was not disappointed, as he had foreseen that the wealth of the Imberts had been greatly exaggerated. It did not consist of hundreds of millions, nor even tens of millions. Yet it amounted to a very respectable sum, and Lupin expressed his satisfaction.

'Of course,' he said, 'there will be a considerable loss when we come to sell the bonds, as we will have to dispose of them surreptitiously at reduced prices. In the meantime, they will rest quietly in my desk awaiting a propitious moment.'

Arsène saw no reason why he should not go to the Imbert house the next day. But a perusal of the morning papers revealed this startling fact: Ludovic and Gervaise Imbert had disappeared.

When the officers of the law seized the safe and opened it, they found there what Arsène Lupin had left – nothing.

Such are the facts; and I learned the sequel to them, one day, when Arsène Lupin was in a confidential mood. He was pacing to and fro in my room, with a nervous step and a feverish eye that were unusual to him.

'After all,' I said to him, 'it was your most successful venture.'

Without making a direct reply, he said:

'There are some impenetrable secrets connected with that affair; some obscure points that escape my comprehension. For instance: What caused their flight? Why did they not take advantage of the help I unconsciously gave them? It would have been so simple to say: "The hundred millions were in the safe. They are no longer there, because they have been stolen."'

'They lost their nerve.'

'Yes, that is it – they lost their nerve . . . On the other hand, it is true—'

'What is true?'

'Oh! nothing.'

What was the meaning of Lupin's reticence? It was quite obvious that he had not told me everything; there was something he was loath to tell. His conduct puzzled me. It must indeed be a very serious matter to cause such a man as Arsène Lupin even a momentary hesitation. I threw out a few questions at random.

'Have you seen them since?'

'No.'

'And have you never experienced the slightest degree of pity for those unfortunate people?'

'I!' he exclaimed, with a start.

His sudden excitement astonished me. Had I touched him on a sore spot? I continued:

'Of course. If you had not left them alone, they might have been able to face the danger, or, at least, made their escape with full pockets.'

'What do you mean?' he said, indignantly. 'I suppose you have an idea that my soul should be filled with remorse?'

'Call it remorse or regrets – anything you like—'

'They are not worth it.'

'Have you no regrets or remorse for having stolen their fortune?'

'What fortune?'

'The packages of bonds you took from their safe.'

'Oh! I stole their bonds, did I? I deprived them of a portion of their wealth? Is that my crime? Ah! my dear boy, you do not know the truth. You never imagined that those bonds were not worth the paper they were written on. Those bonds were false – they were counterfeit – every one of them – do you understand? THEY WERE COUNTERFEIT!'

I looked at him, astounded.

'Counterfeit! The four or five millions?'

'Yes, counterfeit!' he exclaimed, in a fit of rage. 'Only so many scraps of paper! I couldn't raise a sou on the whole of them! And you ask me if I have any remorse. They are the ones who should have remorse and pity. They played me for a simpleton; and I fell into their trap. I was their latest victim, their most stupid gull!'

He was affected by genuine anger – the result of malice and wounded pride. He continued:

'From start to finish, I got the worst of it. Do you know the part I played in that affair, or rather the part they made me play? That of André Brawford! Yes, my boy, that is the truth, and I never suspected it. It was not until afterwards, on reading the newspapers, that the light finally dawned in my stupid brain. Whilst I was posing as his "saviour", as the gentleman who had risked his life to rescue Mon. Imbert from the clutches of an assassin, they were passing me off as Brawford. Wasn't that splendid? That eccentric individual who had a room on the second floor, that barbarian that was exhibited only at a distance, was Brawford, and Brawford was I! Thanks to me, and to the confidence that I inspired under the name of Brawford, they were enabled to borrow money from the bankers and other money-lenders. Ha! what an experience for a novice! And I swear to you that I shall profit by the lesson!'

He stopped, seized my arm, and said to me, in a tone of exasperation:

'My dear fellow, at this very moment, Gervaise Imbert owes me fifteen hundred francs.'

I could not refrain from laughter, his rage was so grotesque. He was making a mountain out of a molehill. In a moment, he laughed himself, and said:

'Yes, my boy, fifteen hundred francs. You must know that I had not received one sou of my promised salary, and, more than that, she had borrowed from me the sum of fifteen hundred francs. All my youthful savings! And do you know why? To devote the money to charity! I am giving you a straight story. She wanted it for some poor people she was assisting – unknown to her husband. And my hard-earned money was wormed out of me by that silly pretence! Isn't it amusing, *hein*? Arsène Lupin done out of fifteen hundred francs by the fair lady from whom he stole four millions in counterfeit bonds! And what a vast amount of time and patience and cunning I expended to achieve that result! It was the first time in my life that I was played for a fool, and I frankly confess that I was fooled that time to the queen's taste!'

AN UNCONVENTIONAL CONFIDENCE

Lucy Maud Montgomery

The Girl in Black-and-Yellow ran frantically down the grey road under the pines. There was nobody to see her, but she would have run if all Halifax had been looking on. For had she not on the loveliest new hat – a 'creation' in yellow chiffon with big black *choux* – and a dress to match? And was there not a shower coming straight from the hills across the harbour?

Down at the end of the long resinous avenue the Girl saw the shore road, with the pavilion shutting out the view of the harbour's mouth. Below the pavilion, clean-shaven George's Island guarded the town like a sturdy bulldog, and beyond it were the wooded hills, already lost in a mist of rain.

'Oh, I shall be too late,' moaned the Girl. But she held her hat steady with one hand and ran on. If she could only reach the pavilion in time! It was a neck-and-neck race between the rain and the Girl, but the Girl won. Just as she flew out upon the shore road, a tall Young Man came pelting down the latter, and they both dashed up the steps of the pavilion together as the rain swooped down upon them and blotted George's Island and the smoky town and the purple banks of the Eastern Passage from view.

The pavilion was small at the best of times, and just now the rain was beating into it on two sides, leaving only one dry corner.

Into this the Girl moved. She was flushed and triumphant. The Young Man thought that in all his life he had never seen anyone so pretty.

'I'm so glad I didn't get my hat wet,' said the Girl breathlessly, as she straightened it with a careful hand and wondered if she looked very blown and blowsy.

'It would have been a pity,' admitted the Young Man. 'It is a very pretty hat.'

'Pretty!' The Girl looked the scorn her voice expressed. 'Anyone can have a *pretty* hat. Our cook has one. This is a *creation*.'

'Of course,' said the Young Man humbly. 'I ought to have known. But I am very stupid.'

'Well, I suppose a mere man couldn't be expected to understand exactly,' said the Girl graciously.

She smiled at him in a friendly fashion, and he smiled back. The Girl thought that she had never seen such lovely brown eyes before. He could not be a Haligonian. She was sure she knew all the nice young men with brown eyes in Halifax.

'Please sit down,' she said plaintively. 'I'm tired.'

The Young Man smiled again at the idea of his sitting down because the Girl was tired. But he sat down, and so did she, on the only dry seat to be found.

'Goodness knows how long this rain will last,' said the Girl, making herself comfortable and picturesque, 'but I shall stay here until it clears up, if it rains for a week. I will *not* have my hat spoiled. I suppose I shouldn't have put it on. Beatrix said it was going to rain. Beatrix is such a horribly good prophet. I detest people who are good prophets, don't you?'

'I think that they are responsible for all the evils that they predict,' said the Young Man solemnly.

'That is just what I told Beatrix. And I was determined to put on this hat and come out to the park today. I simply *had* to be alone, and I knew I'd be alone out here. Everybody else would be at the football game. By the way, why aren't you there?'

'I wasn't even aware that there was a football game on hand,' said the Young Man, as if he knew he ought to be ashamed of his ignorance, and was.

'Dear me,' said the Girl pityingly. 'Where can you have been not to have heard of it? It's between the Dalhousie team and the Wanderers. Almost everybody here is on the Wanderers' side, because they are Haligonians, but I am not. I like the college boys best. Beatrix says that it is just because of my innate contrariness. Last year I simply screamed myself hoarse with enthusiasm. The Dalhousie team won the trophy.'

'If you are so interested in the game, it is a wonder you didn't go to see it yourself,' said the Young Man boldly.

'Well, I just couldn't,' said the Girl with a sigh. 'If anybody had ever told me that there would be a football game in Halifax, and that I would elect to prowl about by myself in the park instead of going to it, I'd have laughed them to scorn. Even Beatrix would never have dared to prophesy *that*. But you see it has happened. I was too crumpled up in my mind to care about football today. I had to come here and have it out with myself. That is why I put on my hat. I thought, perhaps, I might get through with my mental gymnastics in time to go to the game afterwards. But I didn't. It is just maddening, too. I got this hat and dress on purpose to wear to it. They're black and yellow, you see – the Dalhousie colours. It was my own idea. I was sure it would make a sensation. But I couldn't go to the game and take any interest in it, feeling as I do, could I, now?'

The Young Man said, of course, she couldn't. It was utterly out of the question.

The Girl smiled. Without a smile, she was charming. With a smile, she was adorable.

'I like to have my opinions bolstered up. Do you know, I want to tell you something? May I?'

'You may. I'll never tell anyone as long as I live,' said the Young Man solemnly.

'I don't know you and you don't know me. That is why I want to tell you about it. I *must* tell somebody, and if I told anybody I knew, they'd tell it all over Halifax. It is dreadful to be talking to you like this. Beatrix would have three fits, one after the other, if she saw me. But Beatrix is a slave to conventionality. I glory in discarding it at times. You don't mind, do you?'

'Not at all,' said the Young Man sincerely.

The Girl sighed.

'I have reached that point where I must have a confidant, or go crazy. Once I could tell things to Beatrix. That was before she got engaged. Now she tells everything to *him*. There is no earthly way of preventing her. I've tried them all. So, nowadays, when I get into trouble, I tell it out loud to myself in the glass. It's a relief, you know. But that is no good now. I want to tell it to somebody who can say things back. Will you promise to say things back?'

The Young Man assured her that he would when the proper time came.

'Very well. But please don't look at me while I'm telling you. I'll be sure to blush in places. When Beatrix wants to be particularly aggravating she says I have lost the art of blushing. But that is only her way of putting it, you know. Sometimes I blush dreadfully.'

The Young Man dragged his eyes from the face under the black-and-yellow hat, and fastened them on a crooked pine tree that hung out over the bank.

'Well,' began the Girl, 'the root of the whole trouble is simply this. There is a young man in England. I always think of him as the Creature. He is the son of a man who was Father's especial crony in boyhood, before Father emigrated to Canada. Worse than that, he comes of a family which has contracted a vile habit of marrying into our family. It has come down through the ages so long that it has become chronic. Father left most of his musty traditions in England, but he brought this pet one with him. He and this friend agreed that the latter's son should marry one of Father's daughters. It ought to have been Beatrix – she is the oldest. But Beatrix had a pug nose. So Father settled on me. From my earliest recollection I have been given to understand that just as soon as I grew up there would be a ready-made husband imported from England for me. I was doomed to it from my cradle. Now,' said the Girl, with a tragic gesture, 'I ask you, could *anything* be more hopelessly, appallingly stupid and devoid of romance than that?'

The Young Man shook his head, but did not look at her.

'It's pretty bad,' he admitted.

'You see,' said the Girl pathetically, 'the shadow of it has been over my whole life. Of course, when I was a very little girl I didn't mind it so much. It was such a long way off and lots of things might happen. The Creature might run away with some other girl – or I might have the smallpox – or Beatrix's nose might be straight when she grew up. And if Beatrix's nose were straight she'd be a great deal prettier than I am. But nothing did happen – and her nose is puggier than ever. Then when I grew up things were horrid. I never could have a single little bit of fun. And Beatrix had such a good time! She had scores of lovers in spite of her nose. To be sure, she's engaged now – and he's a horrid, faddy little creature. But he is her own choice. She wasn't told that there was a man in England whom she must marry by and by, when he got sufficiently reconciled to the idea to come and ask her. Oh, it makes me furious!'

'Is – is there – anyone else?' asked the Young Man hesitatingly.

'Oh, dear, no. How could there be? Why, you know, I couldn't have the tiniest flirtation with another man when I was as good as engaged to the Creature. That is one of my grievances. Just think how much fun I've missed! I used to rage to Beatrix about it, but she would tell me that I ought to be thankful to have the chance of making such a good match – the Creature is rich, you know, and clever. As if I cared how clever or rich he is! Beatrix made me so cross that I gave up saying anything and sulked by myself. So they think I'm quite reconciled to it, but I'm not.'

'He might be very nice after all,' suggested the Young Man.

'*Nice*! That isn't the point. Oh, don't you see? But no, you're a man – you *can't* understand. You must just take my word for it. The whole thing makes me furious. But I haven't told you the worst. The Creature is on his way out to Canada now. He may arrive here at any minute. And they are all so aggravatingly delighted over it.'

'What do you suppose *he* feels like?' asked the Young Man reflectively.

'Well,' said the Girl frankly, 'I've been too much taken up with my own feelings to worry about his. But I daresay they are pretty much like mine. He must loathe and detest the very thought of me.'

'Oh, I don't think he does,' said the Young Man gravely.

'Don't you? Well, what do you suppose he *does* think of it all? You ought to understand the man's part of it better than I can.'

'There's as much difference in men as in women,' said the Young Man in an impersonal tone. 'I may be right or wrong, you see, but I imagine he would feel something like this: from boyhood he has understood that away out in Canada there is a little girl growing up who is some day to be his wife. She becomes his boyish ideal of all that is good and true. He pictures her as beautiful and winsome and sweet. She is his heart's lady, and the thought of her abides with him as a safeguard and an inspiration. For her sake he resolves to make the most of himself, and live a clean, loyal life. When she comes to him she must find his heart fit to receive her. There is never a time in all his life when the dream of her does not gleam before him as of a star to which he may aspire with all reverence and love.'

The Young Man stopped abruptly, and looked at the Girl. She bent forward with shining eyes, and touched his hand.

'You are splendid,' she said softly. 'If he thought so – but no – I am sure he doesn't. He's just coming out here like a martyr going to the stake. He knows he will be expected to propose to me when he gets here. And he knows that I know it too. And *he* knows and *I* know that I will be expected to say my very prettiest "yes".'

'But are you going to say it?' asked the Young Man anxiously.

The Girl leaned forward. 'No. That is my secret. I am going to say a most emphatic "no".'

'But won't your family make an awful row?'

'Of course. But I rather enjoy a row now and then. It stirs up one's grey matter so nicely. I came out here this afternoon and thought the whole affair over from beginning to end. And I have determined to say "no".'

'Oh, I wouldn't make it so irreconcilable as that,' said the Young Man lightly. 'I'd leave a loophole of escape. You see, if you were to like him a little better than you expect, it would be awkward to have committed yourself by a rash vow to saying "no", wouldn't it?'

'I suppose it would,' said the Girl thoughtfully, 'but then, you know, I won't change my mind.'

'It's just as well to be on the safe side,' said the Young Man.

The Girl got up. The rain was over and the sun was coming out through the mists.

'Perhaps you are right,' she said. 'So I'll just resolve that I will say "no" if I don't want to say "yes". That really amounts to the same thing, you know. Thank you so much for letting me tell you all about it. It must have bored you terribly, but it has done me so much good. I feel quite calm and rational now, and can go home and behave myself. Goodbye.'

'Goodbye,' said the Young Man gravely. He stood on the pavilion and watched the Girl out of sight beyond the pines.

When the Girl got home she was told that the Dalhousie team had won the game, eight to four. The Girl dragged her hat off and waved it joyously.

'What a shame I wasn't there! They'd have gone mad over my dress.'

But the next item of information crushed her. The Creature had arrived. He had called that afternoon, and was coming to dinner that night.

'How fortunate,' said the Girl, as she went to her room, 'that I relieved my mind to that Young Man out in the park today. If I had come back with all that pent-up feeling seething within me and heard this news right on top of it all, I might have flown into a thousand pieces. What lovely brown eyes he had! I do dote on brown eyes. The Creature will be sure to have fishy blue ones.'

When the Girl went down to meet the Creature she found herself confronted by the Young Man. For the first, last and only time in her life, the Girl had not a word to say. But her family thought her confusion very natural and pretty. They really had not expected her to behave so well. As for the Young Man, his manner was flawless.

Toward the end of the dinner, when the Girl was beginning to recover herself, he turned to her.

'You know I promised never to tell,' he said.

'Be sure you don't, then,' said the Girl meekly.

'But aren't you glad you left the loophole?' he persisted.

The Girl smiled down into her lap.

'Perhaps,' she said.

VEROTCHKA

Anton Chekhov

Ivan Alexeyitch Ognev remembers how on that August evening he opened the glass door with a rattle and went out on to the verandah. He was wearing a light Inverness cape and a wide-brimmed straw hat, the very one that was lying with his top-boots in the dust under his bed. In one hand he had a big bundle of books and notebooks, in the other a thick knotted stick.

Behind the door, holding the lamp to show the way, stood the master of the house, Kuznetsov, a bald old man with a long grey beard, in a snow-white piqué jacket. The old man was smiling cordially and nodding his head.

'Good-bye, old fellow!' said Ognev.

Kuznetsov put the lamp on a little table and went out to the verandah. Two long narrow shadows moved down the steps towards the flower-beds, swayed to and fro and leaned their heads on the trunks of the lime-trees.

'Good-bye and once more thank you, my dear fellow!' said Ivan Alexeyitch. 'Thank you for your welcome, for your kindness, for your affection . . . I shall never forget your hospitality as long as I live. You are so good, and your daughter is so good, and everyone here is so kind, so good-humoured and friendly . . . Such a splendid set of people that I don't know how to say what I feel!'

From excess of feeling and under the influence of the home-made wine he had just drunk, Ognev talked in a singing voice like a divinity student, and was so touched that he expressed his feelings not so much by words as by the blinking of his eyes and the twitching of his shoulders. Kuznetsov, who had also drunk a good deal and was touched, craned forward to the young man and kissed him.

'I've grown as fond of you as if I were your dog,' Ognev went on. 'I've been turning up here almost every day; I've stayed the night a dozen times. It's dreadful to think of all the home-made wine I've drunk. And thank you most of all for your co-operation and help. Without you I should have been busy here over my statistics till October. I shall put in my preface: "I think it my duty to express my gratitude to the President of the District Zemstvo of N—, Kuznetsov, for his kind co-operation." There is a brilliant future before statistics! My humble respects to Vera Gavrilovna, and tell the doctors, both the lawyers and your secretary, that I shall never forget their help! And now, old fellow, let us embrace one another and kiss for the last time!'

Ognev, limp with emotion, kissed the old man once more and began going down the steps. On the last step he looked round and asked: 'Shall we meet again some day?'

'God knows!' said the old man. 'Most likely not!'

'Yes, that's true! Nothing will tempt you to Petersburg and I am never likely to turn up in this district again. Well, good-bye!'

'You had better leave the books behind!' Kuznetsov called after him. 'You don't want to drag such a weight with you. I would send them by a servant to-morrow!'

But Ognev was rapidly walking away from the house and was not listening. His heart, warmed by the wine, was brimming over with good-humour, friendliness and sadness. He walked along thinking how frequently one met with good people, and what a pity it was that nothing was left of those meetings but memories. At times one catches a glimpse of cranes on the horizon, and a faint gust of wind brings their plaintive, ecstatic cry, and a minute later, however greedily one scans the blue distance, one cannot see a speck nor catch a sound; and like that, people with their faces and their words flit through our lives and are drowned in the past, leaving nothing except faint traces in the memory. Having been in the N— District from the early spring, and having been almost every day at the friendly Kuznetsovs', Ivan Alexeyitch had become as much at home with the old man, his daughter and the servants as though they were his own people; he had grown familiar with the whole house to the smallest detail, with the cosy verandah, the windings of the avenues, the silhouettes of the trees over the kitchen and the bath-house; but as soon as he was out of the gate all this would be changed to memory and would lose its meaning as reality for ever, and in a year or two all these dear images would grow as dim in his consciousness as stories he had read or things he had imagined.

'Nothing in life is so precious as people!' Ognev thought in his emotion, as he strode along the avenue to the gate. 'Nothing!'

It was warm and still in the garden. There was a scent of the mignonette, of the tobacco-plants and of the heliotrope, which were not yet over in the flower-beds. The spaces between the bushes and the tree-trunks were filled with a fine soft mist soaked through and through with moonlight, and, as Ognev long remembered, coils of mist that looked like phantoms slowly but perceptibly followed one another across the avenue. The moon stood high above the garden, and below it transparent patches of mist were floating eastward. The whole world seemed to consist of nothing but black silhouettes and wandering white shadows. Ognev, seeing the mist on a moonlight August evening almost for the first time in his life, imagined he was seeing, not nature, but a stage effect in which unskilful workmen, trying to light up the garden with white Bengal fire, hid behind the bushes and let off clouds of white smoke together with the light.

When Ognev reached the garden gate a dark shadow moved away from the low fence and came towards him.

'Vera Gavrilovna!' he said, delighted. 'You here? And I have been looking everywhere for you; wanted to say good-bye . . . Good-bye; I am going away!'

'So early? Why, it's only eleven o'clock.'

'Yes, it's time I was off. I have a four-mile walk and then my packing. I must be up early to-morrow.'

Before Ognev stood Kuznetsov's daughter Vera, a girl of one-and-twenty, as usual melancholy, carelessly dressed and attractive. Girls who are dreamy and spend whole days lying down, lazily reading whatever they come across, who are bored and melancholy, are usually careless in their dress. To those of them who have been endowed by nature with taste and an instinct of beauty, the slight carelessness adds a special charm. When Ognev later on remembered her, he could not picture pretty Verotchka except in a full blouse which was crumpled in deep folds at the belt and yet did not touch her waist; without her hair done up high and a curl that had come loose from it on her forehead; without the knitted red shawl with ball fringe at the edge which hung disconsolately on Vera's shoulders in the evenings, like a flag on a windless day, and in the daytime lay about, crushed up, in the hall near the men's hats or on a box in the dining-room, where the old cat did not hesitate to sleep on it. This shawl and the folds of her blouse suggested a feeling of freedom and laziness, of good-nature and sitting at home. Perhaps because Vera attracted Ognev he saw in every frill and button something warm, naïve, cosy, something nice and poetical, just what is lacking in cold, insincere women that have no instinct for beauty.

Verotchka had a good figure, a regular profile and beautiful curly hair. Ognev, who had seen few women in his life, thought her a beauty.

'I am going away,' he said as he took leave of her at the gate. 'Don't remember evil against me! Thank you for everything!'

In the same singing divinity student's voice in which he had talked to her father, with the same blinking and twitching of his shoulders, he began thanking Vera for her hospitality, kindness and friendliness.

'I've written about you in every letter to my mother,' he said. 'If everyone were like you and your dad, what a jolly place the world would be! You are such a splendid set of people! All such genuine, friendly people with no nonsense about you.'

'Where are you going to now?' asked Vera.

'I am going now to my mother's at Oryol; I shall be a fortnight with her, and then back to Petersburg and work.'

'And then?'

'And then? I shall work all the winter and in the spring go somewhere into the provinces again to collect material. Well, be happy, live a hundred years . . . don't remember evil against me. We shall not see each other again.'

Ognev stooped down and kissed Vera's hand. Then, in silent emotion, he straightened his cape, shifted his bundle of books to a more comfortable position, paused and said:

'What a lot of mist!'

'Yes. Have you left anything behind?'

'No, I don't think so . . .'

For some seconds Ognev stood in silence, then he moved clumsily towards the gate and went out of the garden.

'Stay; I'll see you as far as our wood,' said Vera, following him out.

They walked along the road. Now the trees did not obscure the view, and one could see the sky and the distance. As though covered with a veil all nature was hidden in a transparent, colourless haze through which her beauty peeped gaily; where the mist was thicker and whiter it lay heaped unevenly about the stones, stalks and bushes or drifted in coils over the road, clung close to the earth and seemed trying not to conceal the view. Through the haze they could see all the road as far as the wood, with dark ditches at the sides and tiny bushes which grew in the ditches and caught the straying wisps of mist. Half a mile from the gate they saw the dark patch of Kuznetsov's wood.

'Why has she come with me? I shall have to see her back,' thought Ognev, but looking at her profile he gave a friendly smile and said: 'One doesn't want to go away in such lovely weather. It's quite a romantic evening, with the moon, the stillness and all the etceteras. Do you know, Vera Gavrilovna, here I have lived twenty-nine years in the world and never had a romance. No romantic episode in my whole life, so that I only know by hearsay of rendezvous, "avenues of sighs" and kisses. It's not normal! In town, when one sits in one's lodgings, one does not notice the blank, but here in the fresh air one feels it . . . One resents it!'

'Why is it?'

'I don't know. I suppose I've never had time, or perhaps it was I have never met women who . . . In fact, I have very few acquaintances and never go anywhere.'

For some three hundred paces the young people walked on in silence. Ognev kept glancing at Verotchka's bare head and shawl, and days of spring and summer rose to his mind one after another. It had been a period when far from his grey Petersburg lodgings, enjoying the friendly warmth of kind people, nature and the work he loved, he had not had time to notice how the sunsets followed the glow of dawn, and how, one after another foretelling the end of summer, first the nightingale ceased singing, then the quail, then a little later the landrail. The days slipped by unnoticed, so that life must have been happy and easy. He began calling aloud how reluctantly he, poor and unaccustomed to change of scene and society, had come at the end of April to the N— District, where he had expected dreariness, loneliness and indifference to statistics, which he considered was now the foremost among the sciences. When he arrived on an April morning at the little town of N— he had put up at the inn kept by Ryabuhin, the Old Believer, where for twenty kopecks a day they had given him a light, clean room on condition that he should not smoke indoors. After resting and finding who was the president of the District Zemstvo, he had set off at once on foot to Kuznetsov. He had to walk three miles through lush meadows and young copses. Larks were hovering in the clouds, filling the air with silvery notes, and rooks flapping their wings with sedate dignity floated over the green cornland.

'Good heavens!' Ognev had thought in wonder; 'can it be that there's always air like this to breathe here, or is this scent only to-day, in honour of my coming?'

Expecting a cold business-like reception, he went in to Kuznetsov's diffidently, looking up from under his eyebrows and shyly pulling his beard. At first Kuznetsov wrinkled up his brows and could not understand what use the Zemstvo could be to the young man and his statistics; but when the latter explained at length what was material for statistics and how such material was collected, Kuznetsov brightened, smiled and with childish curiosity began looking at his notebooks. On the evening of the same day Ivan Alexeyitch was already sitting at supper with the Kuznetsovs, was rapidly becoming exhilarated by their strong home-made wine, and looking at the calm faces and lazy movements of his new acquaintances, felt all over that sweet, drowsy indolence which makes one want to sleep and stretch and smile; while his new acquaintances looked at him good-naturedly and asked him whether his father and mother were living, how much he earned a month, how often he went to the theatre . . .

Ognev recalled his expeditions about the neighbourhood, the picnics, the fishing parties, the visit of the whole party to the convent to see the Mother Superior Marfa, who had given each of the visitors a bead purse; he recalled the hot, endless typically Russian arguments in which the opponents, spluttering and banging the table with their fists, misunderstand and interrupt one another, unconsciously contradict themselves at every phrase, continually change the subject, and after arguing for two or three hours, laugh and say: 'Goodness knows what we have been arguing about! Beginning with one thing and going on to another!'

'And do you remember how the doctor and you and I rode to Shestovo?' said Ivan Alexeyitch to Vera as they reached the copse. 'It was there that the crazy saint met us: I gave him a five-kopeck piece, and he crossed himself three times and flung it into the rye. Good heavens! I am carrying away such a mass of memories that if I could gather them together into a whole it would make a good nugget of gold! I don't understand why clever, perceptive people crowd into Petersburg and Moscow and don't come here. Is there more truth and freedom in the Nevsky and in the big damp houses than here? Really, the idea of artists, scientific men and journalists all living crowded together in furnished rooms has always seemed to me a mistake.'

Twenty paces from the copse the road was crossed by a small narrow bridge with posts at the corners, which had always served as a resting-place for the Kuznetsovs and their guests on their evening walks. From there those who liked could mimic the forest echo, and one could see the road vanish in the dark woodland track.

'Well, here is the bridge!' said Ognev. 'Here you must turn back.'

Vera stopped and drew a breath.

'Let us sit down,' she said, sitting down on one of the posts. 'People generally sit down when they say good-bye before starting on a journey.'

Ognev settled himself beside her on his bundle of books and went on talking. She was breathless from the walk, and was looking, not at Ivan Alexeyitch, but away into the distance so that he could not see her face.

'And what if we meet in ten years' time?' he said. 'What shall we be like then? You will be by then the respectable mother of a family, and I shall be the author of some weighty statistical work of no use to anyone, as thick as forty thousand such works. We shall meet and think of old days... Now we are conscious of the present; it absorbs and excites us, but when we meet we shall not remember the day, nor the month, nor even the year in which we saw each other for the last time on this bridge. You will be changed, perhaps... Tell me, will you be different?'

Vera started and turned her face towards him.

'What?' she asked.

'I asked you just now...'

'Excuse me, I did not hear what you were saying.'

Only then Ognev noticed a change in Vera. She was pale, breathing fast, and the tremor in her breathing affected her hands and lips and head, and not one curl as usual, but two, came loose and fell on her forehead... Evidently she avoided looking him in the face, and, trying to mask her emotion, at one moment fingered her collar, which seemed to be rasping her neck, at another pulled her red shawl from one shoulder to the other.

'I am afraid you are cold,' said Ognev. 'It's not at all wise to sit in the mist. Let me see you back *nach-haus*.'

Vera sat mute.

'What is the matter?' asked Ognev, with a smile. 'You sit silent and don't answer my questions. Are you cross, or don't you feel well?'

Vera pressed the palm of her hand to the cheek nearest to Ognev, and then abruptly jerked it away.

'An awful position!' she murmured, with a look of pain on her face. 'Awful!'

'How is it awful?' asked Ognev, shrugging his shoulders and not concealing his surprise. 'What's the matter?'

Still breathing hard and twitching her shoulders, Vera turned her back to him, looked at the sky for half a minute and said:

'There is something I must say to you, Ivan Alexeyitch . . .'

'I am listening.'

'It may seem strange to you . . . You will be surprised, but I don't care . . .'

Ognev shrugged his shoulders once more and prepared himself to listen.

'You see . . .' Verotchka began, bowing her head and fingering a ball on the fringe of her shawl. 'You see . . . this is what I wanted to tell you . . . You'll think it strange . . . and silly, but I . . . can't bear it any longer.'

Vera's words died away in an indistinct mutter and were suddenly cut short by tears. The girl hid her face in her handkerchief, bent lower than ever and wept bitterly. Ivan Alexeyitch cleared his throat in confusion and looked about him hopelessly, at his wits' end, not knowing what to say or do. Being unused to the sight of tears, he felt his own eyes, too, beginning to smart.

'Well, what next!' he muttered helplessly. 'Vera Gavrilovna, what's this for, I should like to know? My dear girl, are you . . . are you ill? Or has someone been nasty to you? Tell me, perhaps I could, so to say . . . help you . . .'

When, trying to console her, he ventured cautiously to remove her hands from her face, she smiled at him through her tears and said:

'I . . . love you!'

These words, so simple and ordinary, were uttered in ordinary human language, but Ognev, in acute embarrassment, turned away from Vera, and got up, while his confusion was followed by terror.

The sad, warm, sentimental mood induced by leave-taking and the home-made wine suddenly vanished, and gave place to an acute and unpleasant feeling of awkwardness. He felt an inward revulsion; he looked askance at Vera, and now that by declaring her love for him she had cast off the aloofness which so adds to a woman's charm, she seemed to him, as it were, shorter, plainer, more ordinary.

'What's the meaning of it?' he thought with horror. 'But I . . . do I love her or not? That's the question!'

And she breathed easily and freely now that the worst and most difficult thing was said. She, too, got up, and looking Ivan Alexeyitch straight in the face, began talking rapidly, warmly, irrepressibly.

As a man suddenly panic-stricken cannot afterwards remember the succession of sounds accompanying the catastrophe that overwhelmed him, so Ognev cannot remember Vera's words and phrases. He can only recall the meaning of what she said, and the sensation her words evoked in him. He remembers her voice, which seemed stifled and husky with emotion, and the extraordinary music and passion of her intonation. Laughing, crying with tears glistening on her eyelashes, she told him that from the first day of their acquaintance he had struck her by his originality, his intelligence, his kind intelligent eyes, by his work and objects in life; that she loved him passionately, deeply, madly; that when coming into the house from the garden in the summer she saw his cape in the hall or heard his voice in the distance, she felt a cold shudder at her heart, a foreboding of happiness; even his slightest jokes had made her laugh; in every figure in his note-books she saw something extraordinarily wise and grand; his knotted stick seemed to her more beautiful than the trees.

The copse and the wisps of mist and the black ditches at the side of the road seemed hushed listening to her, whilst something strange and unpleasant was passing in Ognev's heart . . . Telling him of her love, Vera was enchantingly beautiful; she spoke eloquently and passionately, but he felt neither pleasure nor gladness, as he would have liked to; he felt nothing but compassion for Vera, pity and regret that a good girl should be distressed on his account. Whether he was affected by generalizations from reading or by the insuperable habit of looking at things objectively, which so often hinders people from living, but Vera's ecstasies and suffering struck him as affected, not to be taken seriously, and at the same time rebellious feeling whispered to him that all he was hearing and seeing now, from the point of view of nature and personal happiness, was more important than any statistics and books and truths . . . And he raged and blamed himself, though he did not understand exactly where he was in fault.

To complete his embarrassment, he was absolutely at a loss what to say, and yet something he must say. To say bluntly, 'I don't love you,' was beyond him, and he could not bring himself to say, 'Yes,' because however much he rummaged in his heart he could not find one spark of feeling in it . . .

He was silent, and she meanwhile was saying that for her there was no greater happiness than to see him, to follow him wherever he liked this very moment, to be his wife and helper, and that if he went away from her she would die of misery.

'I cannot stay here!' she said, wringing her hands. 'I am sick of the house and this wood and the air. I cannot bear the everlasting peace and aimless life, I can't endure our colourless, pale people, who are all as like one another as two drops of water! They are all good-natured and warm-hearted because they are all well-fed and know nothing of struggle or suffering . . . I want to be in those big damp houses where people suffer, embittered by work and need . . .'

And this, too, seemed to Ognev affected and not to be taken seriously. When Vera had finished he still did not know what to say, but it was impossible to be silent, and he muttered:

'Vera Gavrilovna, I am very grateful to you, though I feel I've done nothing to deserve such . . . feeling . . . on your part. Besides, as an honest man I ought to tell you that . . . happiness depends on equality – that is, when both parties are . . . equally in love . . .'

But he was immediately ashamed of his mutterings and ceased. He felt that his face at that moment looked stupid, guilty, blank, that it was strained and affected . . . Vera must have been able to read the truth on his countenance, for she suddenly became grave, turned pale and bent her head.

'You must forgive me,' Ognev muttered, not able to endure the silence. 'I respect you so much that . . . it pains me . . .'

Vera turned sharply and walked rapidly homewards. Ognev followed her.

'No, don't!' said Vera, with a wave of her hand. 'Don't come; I can go alone.'

'Oh, yes . . . I must see you home anyway.'

Whatever Ognev said, it all to the last word struck him as loathsome and flat. The feeling of guilt grew greater at every step. He raged inwardly, clenched his fists and cursed his coldness and his stupidity with women. Trying to stir his feelings, he looked at Verotchka's beautiful figure, at her hair and the traces of her little feet on the dusty road; he remembered her words and her tears, but all that only touched his heart and did not quicken his pulse.

'Ach! one can't force oneself to love,' he assured himself, and at the same time he thought, 'But shall I ever fall in love without? I am nearly thirty! I have never met anyone better than Vera and I never shall . . . Oh, this premature old age! Old age at thirty!'

Vera walked on in front more and more rapidly, without looking back at him or raising her head. It seemed to him that sorrow had made her thinner and narrower in the shoulders.

'I can imagine what's going on in her heart now!' he thought, looking at her back. 'She must be ready to die with shame and mortification! My God, there's so much life, poetry and meaning in it that it would move a stone, and I . . . I am stupid and absurd!'

At the gate Vera stole a glance at him, and, shrugging and wrapping her shawl round her walked rapidly away down the avenue.

Ivan Alexeyitch was left alone. Going back to the copse, he walked slowly, continually standing still and looking round at the gate with an expression in his whole figure that suggested that he could not believe his own memory. He looked for Vera's footprints on the road, and could not believe that the girl who had so attracted him had just declared her love, and that he had so clumsily and bluntly 'refused' her. For the first time in his life it was his lot to learn by experience how little that a man does depends on his own will, and to suffer in his own person the feelings of a decent kindly man who has against his will caused his neighbour cruel, undeserved anguish.

His conscience tormented him, and when Vera disappeared he felt as though he had lost something very precious, something very near and dear which he could never find again. He felt that with Vera a part of his youth had slipped away from him, and that the moments which he had passed through so fruitlessly would never be repeated.

When he reached the bridge he stopped and sank into thought. He wanted to discover the reason of his strange coldness. That it was due to something within him and not outside himself was clear to him. He frankly acknowledged to himself that it was not the intellectual coldness of which clever people so often boast, not the coldness of a conceited fool, but simply impotence of soul, incapacity for being moved by beauty, premature old age brought on by education, his casual existence, struggling for a livelihood, his homeless life in lodgings. From the bridge he walked slowly, as it were reluctantly, into the wood. Here, where in the dense black darkness glaring patches of moonlight gleamed here and there, where he felt nothing except his thoughts, he longed passionately to regain what he had lost.

And Ivan Alexeyitch remembers that he went back again. Urging himself on with his memories, forcing himself to picture Vera, he strode rapidly towards the garden. There was no mist by then along the road or in the garden, and the bright moon looked down from the sky as though it had just been washed; only the eastern sky was dark and misty . . . Ognev remembers his cautious steps, the dark windows, the heavy scent of heliotrope and mignonette. His old friend Karo, wagging his tail amicably, came up to him and sniffed his hand. This was the one living creature who saw him walk two or three times round the house, stand near Vera's dark window and with a deep sigh and a wave of his hand walk out of the garden.

An hour later he was in the town, and, worn out and exhausted, leaned his body and hot face against the gatepost of the inn as he knocked at the gate. Somewhere in the town a dog barked sleepily, and as though in response to his knock, someone clanged the hour on an iron plate near the church.

'You prowl about at night,' grumbled his host, the Old Believer, opening the door to him, in a long nightgown like a woman's. 'You had better be saying your prayers instead of prowling about.'

When Ivan Alexeyitch reached his room he sank on the bed and gazed a long, long time at the light. Then he tossed his head and began packing.

THE DEVOTED FRIEND

Oscar Wilde

One morning the old Water-rat put his head out of his hole. He had bright beady eyes and stiff grey whiskers and his tail was like a long bit of black India-rubber. The little ducks were swimming about in the pond, looking just like a lot of yellow canaries, and their mother, who was pure white with real red legs, was trying to teach them how to stand on their heads in the water.

'You will never be in the best society unless you can stand on your heads,' she kept saying to them; and every now and then she showed them how it was done. But the little ducks paid no attention to her. They were so young that they did not know what an advantage it is to be in society at all.

'What disobedient children!' cried the old Water-rat; 'they really deserve to be drowned.'

'Nothing of the kind,' answered the Duck, 'every one must make a beginning, and parents cannot be too patient.'

'Ah! I know nothing about the feelings of parents,' said the Water-rat; 'I am not a family man. In fact, I have never been married, and I never intend to be. Love is all very well in its way, but friendship is much higher. Indeed, I know of nothing in the world that is either nobler or rarer than a devoted friendship.'

'And what, pray, is your idea of the duties of a devoted friend?'

asked a Green Linnet, who was sitting in a willow-tree hard by, and had overheard the conversation.

'Yes, that is just what I want to know,' said the Duck; and she swam away to the end of the pond, and stood upon her head, in order to give her children a good example.

'What a silly question!' cried the Water-rat. 'I should expect my devoted friend to be devoted to me, of course.'

'And what would you do in return?' said the little bird, swinging upon a silver spray, and flapping his tiny wings.

'I don't understand you,' answered the Water-rat.

'Let me tell you a story on the subject,' said the Linnet.

'Is the story about me?' asked the Water-rat. 'If so, I will listen to it, for I am extremely fond of fiction.'

'It is applicable to you,' answered the Linnet; and he flew down, and alighting upon the bank, he told the story of The Devoted Friend.

'Once upon a time,' said the Linnet, 'there was an honest little fellow named Hans.'

'Was he very distinguished?' asked the Water-rat.

'No,' answered the Linnet, 'I don't think he was distinguished at all, except for his kind heart, and his funny round good-humoured face. He lived in a tiny cottage all by himself, and every day he worked in his garden. In all the country-side there was no garden so lovely as his. Sweet-william grew there, and Gilly-flowers, and Shepherds'-purses, and Fair-maids of France. There were damask Roses, and yellow Roses, lilac Crocuses, and gold, purple Violets and white. Columbine and Ladysmock, Marjoram and Wild Basil, the Cowslip and the Flower-de-luce, the Daffodil and the Clove-Pink bloomed or blossomed in their proper order as the months went by, one flower taking another flower's place, so that there were always beautiful things to look at, and pleasant odours to smell.

'Little Hans had a great many friends, but the most devoted friend of all was big Hugh the Miller. Indeed, so devoted was the rich Miller to little Hans, that he would never go by his garden without leaning over the wall and plucking a large nosegay, or a handful of sweet herbs, or filling his pockets with plums and cherries if it was the fruit season.

'"Real friends should have everything in common," the Miller used to say, and little Hans nodded and smiled, and felt very proud of having a friend with such noble ideas.

'Sometimes, indeed, the neighbours thought it strange that the rich Miller never gave little Hans anything in return, though he had a hundred sacks of flour stored away in his mill, and six milch cows, and a large flock of woolly sheep; but Hans never troubled his head about these things, and nothing gave him greater pleasure than to listen to all the wonderful things the Miller used to say about the unselfishness of true friendship.

'So little Hans worked away in his garden. During the spring, the summer and the autumn he was very happy, but when the winter came, and he had no fruit or flowers to bring to the market, he suffered a good deal from cold and hunger, and often had to go to bed without any supper but a few dried pears or some hard nuts. In the winter, also, he was extremely lonely, as the Miller never came to see him then.

'"There is no good in my going to see little Hans as long as the snow lasts," the Miller used to say to his wife, "for when people are in trouble they should be left alone, and not be bothered by visitors. That at least is my idea about friendship, and I am sure I am right. So I shall wait till the spring comes, and then I shall pay him a visit, and he will be able to give me a large basket of primroses and that will make him so happy."

'"You are certainly very thoughtful about others," answered the

Wife, as she sat in her comfortable armchair by the big pinewood fire; "very thoughtful indeed. It is quite a treat to hear you talk about friendship. I am sure the clergyman himself could not say such beautiful things as you do, though he does live in a three-storied house, and wear a gold ring on his little finger."

'"But could we not ask little Hans up here?" said the Miller's youngest son. "If poor Hans is in trouble I will give him half my porridge, and show him my white rabbits."

'"What a silly boy you are!" cried the Miller; "I really don't know what is the use of sending you to school. You seem not to learn anything. Why, if little Hans came up here, and saw our warm fire, and our good supper, and our great cask of red wine, he might get envious, and envy is a most terrible thing, and would spoil anybody's nature. I certainly will not allow Hans' nature to be spoiled. I am his best friend, and I will always watch over him, and see that he is not led into any temptations. Besides, if Hans came here, he might ask me to let him have some flour on credit, and that I could not do. Flour is one thing, and friendship is another, and they should not be confused. Why, the words are spelt differently, and mean quite different things. Everybody can see that."

'"How well you talk!" said the Miller's Wife, pouring herself out a large glass of warm ale; "really I feel quite drowsy. It is just like being in church."

'"Lots of people act well," answered the Miller; "but very few people talk well, which shows that talking is much the more difficult thing of the two, and much the finer thing also"; and he looked sternly across the table at his little son, who felt so ashamed of himself that he hung his head down, and grew quite scarlet, and began to cry into his tea. However, he was so young that you must excuse him.'

'Is that the end of the story?' asked the Water-rat.

'Certainly not,' answered the Linnet, 'that is the beginning.'

'Then you are quite behind the age,' said the Water-rat. 'Every good story-teller nowadays starts with the end, and then goes on to the beginning, and concludes with the middle. That is the new method. I heard all about it the other day from a critic who was walking round the pond with a young man. He spoke of the matter at great length, and I am sure he must have been right, for he had blue spectacles and a bald head, and whenever the young man made any remark, he always answered "Pooh!" But pray go on with your story. I like the Miller immensely. I have all kinds of beautiful sentiments myself, so there is a great sympathy between us.'

'Well,' said the Linnet, hopping now on one leg and now on the other, 'as soon as the winter was over, and the primroses began to open their pale yellow stars, the Miller said to his wife that he would go down and see little Hans.

'"Why, what a good heart you have!" cried his Wife; "you are always thinking of others. And mind you take the big basket with you for the flowers."

'So the Miller tied the sails of the windmill together with a strong iron chain, and went down the hill with the basket on his arm.

'"Good morning, little Hans," said the Miller.

'"Good morning," said Hans, leaning on his spade, and smiling from ear to ear.

'"And how have you been all the winter?" said the Miller.

'"Well, really," cried Hans, "it is very good of you to ask, very good indeed. I am afraid I had rather a hard time of it, but now the spring has come, and I am quite happy, and all my flowers are doing well."

'"We often talked of you during the winter, Hans," said the Miller, "and wondered how you were getting on."

"'That was kind of you," said Hans; "I was half afraid you had forgotten me."

"'Hans, I am surprised at you," said the Miller; "friendship never forgets. That is the wonderful thing about it, but I am afraid you don't understand the poetry of life. How lovely your primroses are looking, by-the-bye!"

"'They are certainly very lovely," said Hans, "and it is a most lucky thing for me that I have so many. I am going to bring them into the market and sell them to the Burgomaster's daughter, and buy back my wheelbarrow with the money."

"'Buy back your wheelbarrow? You don't mean to say you have sold it? What a very stupid thing to do!"

"'Well, the fact is," said Hans, "that I was obliged to. You see the winter was a very bad time for me, and I really had no money at all to buy bread with. So I first sold the silver buttons off my Sunday coat, and then I sold my silver chain, and then I sold my big pipe, and at last I sold my wheelbarrow. But I am going to buy them all back again now."

"'Hans," said the Miller, "I will give you my wheelbarrow. It is not in very good repair; indeed, one side is gone, and there is something wrong with the wheel-spokes; but in spite of that I will give it to you. I know it is very generous of me, and a great many people would think me extremely foolish for parting with it, but I am not like the rest of the world. I think that generosity is the essence of friendship, and, besides, I have got a new wheelbarrow for myself. Yes, you may set your mind at ease, I will give you my wheelbarrow."

"'Well, really, that is generous of you," said little Hans, and his funny round face glowed all over with pleasure. "I can easily put it in repair, as I have a plank of wood in the house."

"'A plank of wood!" said the Miller; "why, that is just what I want for the roof of my barn. There is a very large hole in it, and the corn will all get damp if I don't stop it up. How lucky you mentioned it! It is quite remarkable how one good action always breeds another. I have given you my wheelbarrow, and now you are going to give me your plank. Of course, the wheelbarrow is worth far more than the plank, but true friendship never notices things like that. Pray get it at once, and I will set to work at my barn this very day."

"'Certainly,' cried little Hans, and he ran into the shed and dragged the plank out.

"'It is not a very big plank,' said the Miller, looking at it, "and I am afraid that after I have mended my barn-roof there won't be any left for you to mend the wheelbarrow with; but, of course, that is not my fault. And now, as I have given you my wheelbarrow, I am sure you would like to give me some flowers in return. Here is the basket, and mind you fill it quite full."

"'Quite full?' said little Hans, rather sorrowfully, for it was really a very big basket, and he knew that if he filled it he would have no flowers left for the market and he was very anxious to get his silver buttons back.

"'Well, really,' answered the Miller, "as I have given you my wheelbarrow, I don't think that it is much to ask you for a few flowers. I may be wrong, but I should have thought that friendship, true friendship, was quite free from selfishness of any kind."

"'My dear friend, my best friend,' cried little Hans, "you are welcome to all the flowers in my garden. I would much sooner have your good opinion than my silver buttons, any day"; and he ran and plucked all his pretty primroses, and filled the Miller's basket.

"'Good-bye, little Hans,' said the Miller, as he went up the hill with the plank on his shoulder, and the big basket in his hand.

"'Good-bye,' said little Hans, and he began to dig away quite merrily, he was so pleased about the wheelbarrow.

'The next day he was nailing up some honeysuckle against the porch, when he heard the Miller's voice calling to him from the road. So he jumped off the ladder, and ran down the garden, and looked over the wall.

'There was the Miller with a large sack of flour on his back.

'"Dear little Hans," said the Miller, "would you mind carrying this sack of flour for me to market?"

'"Oh, I am so sorry,' said Hans, 'but I am really very busy to-day. I have got all my creepers to nail up, and all my flowers to water, and all my grass to roll."

'"Well, really," said the Miller, "I think that, considering that I am going to give you my wheelbarrow, it is rather unfriendly of you to refuse."

'"Oh, don't say that," cried little Hans, "I wouldn't be unfriendly for the whole world"; and he ran in for his cap, and trudged off with the big sack on his shoulders.

'It was a very hot day, and the road was terribly dusty, and before Hans had reached the sixth milestone he was so tired that he had to sit down and rest. However, he went on bravely, and at last he reached the market. After he had waited there some time, he sold the sack of flour for a very good price, and then he returned home at once, for he was afraid that if he stopped too late he might meet some robbers on the way.

'"It has certainly been a hard day," said little Hans to himself as he was going to bed, "but I am glad I did not refuse the Miller, for he is my best friend, and, besides, he is going to give me his wheelbarrow."

'Early the next morning the Miller came down to get the money for his sack of flour, but little Hans was so tired that he was still in bed.

'"Upon my word," said the Miller, "you are very lazy. Really,

184

considering that I am going to give you my wheelbarrow, I think you might work harder. Idleness is a great sin, and I certainly don't like any of my friends to be idle or sluggish. You must not mind my speaking quite plainly to you. Of course I should not dream of doing so if I were not your friend. But what is the good of friendship if one cannot say exactly what one means? Anybody can say charming things and try to please and to flatter, but a true friend always says unpleasant things, and does not mind giving pain. Indeed, if he is a really true friend he prefers it, for he knows that then he is doing good."

"'I am very sorry,' said little Hans, rubbing his eyes and pulling off his night-cap, "but I was so tired that I thought I would lie in bed for a little time, and listen to the birds singing. Do you know that I always work better after hearing the birds sing?"

"'Well, I am glad of that,' said the Miller, clapping little Hans on the back, "for I want you to come up to the mill as soon as you are dressed, and mend my barn-roof for me."

'Poor little Hans was very anxious to go and work in his garden, for his flowers had not been watered for two days, but he did not like to refuse the Miller, as he was such a good friend to him.

"'Do you think it would be unfriendly of me if I said I was busy?" he inquired in a shy and timid voice.

"'Well, really,' answered the Miller, "I do not think it is much to ask of you, considering that I am going to give you my wheelbarrow; but of course if you refuse I will go and do it myself."

"'Oh! on no account,' cried little Hans and he jumped out of bed, and dressed himself, and went up to the barn.

'He worked there all day long, till sunset, and at sunset the Miller came to see how he was getting on.

"'Have you mended the hole in the roof yet, little Hans?" cried the Miller in a cheery voice.

'"It is quite mended," answered little Hans, coming down the ladder.

'"Ah!" said the Miller, "there is no work so delightful as the work one does for others."

'"It is certainly a great privilege to hear you talk," answered little Hans, sitting down, and wiping his forehead, "a very great privilege. But I am afraid I shall never have such beautiful ideas as you have."

'"Oh! they will come to you," said the Miller, "but you must take more pains. At present you have only the practice of friendship; some day you will have the theory also."

'"Do you really think I shall?" asked little Hans.

'"I have no doubt of it," answered the Miller, "but now that you have mended the roof, you had better go home and rest, for I want you to drive my sheep to the mountain to-morrow."

'Poor little Hans was afraid to say anything to this, and early the next morning the Miller brought his sheep round to the cottage, and Hans started off with them to the mountain. It took him the whole day to get there and back; and when he returned he was so tired that he went off to sleep in his chair, and did not wake up till it was broad daylight.

'"What a delightful time I shall have in my garden," he said, and he went to work at once.

'But somehow he was never able to look after his flowers at all, for his friend the Miller was always coming round and sending him off on long errands, or getting him to help at the mill. Little Hans was very much distressed at times, as he was afraid his flowers would think he had forgotten them, but he consoled himself by the reflection that the Miller was his best friend. "Besides," he used to say, "he is going to give me his wheelbarrow, and that is an act of pure generosity."

'So little Hans worked away for the Miller, and the Miller said all kinds of beautiful things about friendship, which Hans took down in a note-book, and used to read over at night, for he was a very good scholar.

'Now it happened that one evening little Hans was sitting by his fireside when a loud rap came at the door. It was a very wild night, and the wind was blowing and roaring round the house so terribly that at first he thought it was merely the storm. But a second rap came, and then a third, louder than any of the others.

'"It is some poor traveller," said little Hans to himself, and he ran to the door.

'There stood the Miller with a lantern in one hand and a big stick in the other.

'"Dear little Hans," cried the Miller, "I am in great trouble. My little boy has fallen off a ladder and hurt himself, and I am going for the Doctor. But he lives so far away, and it is such a bad night, that it has just occurred to me that it would be much better if you went instead of me. You know I am going to give you my wheelbarrow, and so, it is only fair that you should do something for me in return."

'"Certainly," cried little Hans, "I take it quite as a compliment your coming to me, and I will start off at once. But you must lend me your lantern, as the night is so dark that I am afraid I might fall into the ditch."

'"I am very sorry," answered the Miller, "but it is my new lantern, and it would be a great loss to me if anything happened to it."

'"Well, never mind, I will do without it," cried little Hans, and he took down his great fur coat, and his warm scarlet cap, and tied a muffler round his throat, and started off.

'What a dreadful storm it was! The night was so black that little Hans could hardly see, and the wind was so strong that he could scarcely stand. However, he was very courageous, and after he had been walking about three hours, he arrived at the Doctor's house, and knocked at the door.

'"Who is there?" cried the Doctor, putting his head out of his bedroom window.

'"Little Hans, Doctor."

'"What do you want, little Hans?"

'"The Miller's son has fallen from a ladder, and has hurt himself, and the Miller wants you to come at once."

'"All right!" said the Doctor; and he ordered his horse, and his big boots, and his lantern, and came downstairs, and rode off in the direction of the Miller's house, little Hans trudging behind him.

'But the storm grew worse and worse, and the rain fell in torrents, and little Hans could not see where he was going, or keep up with the horse. At last he lost his way, and wandered off on the moor, which was a very dangerous place, as it was full of deep holes, and there poor little Hans was drowned. His body was found the next day by some goatherds, floating in a great pool of water, and was brought back by them to the cottage.

'Everybody went to little Hans' funeral, as he was so popular, and the Miller was the chief mourner.

'"As I was his best friend," said the Miller, "it is only fair that I should have the best place"; so he walked at the head of the procession in a long black cloak, and every now and then he wiped his eyes with a big pocket-handkerchief.

'"Little Hans is certainly a great loss to every one," said the Blacksmith, when the funeral was over, and they were all seated comfortably in the inn, drinking spiced wine and eating sweet cakes.

'"A great loss to me at any rate," answered the Miller; "why, I had as good as given him my wheelbarrow, and now I really don't know what to do with it. It is very much in my way at home, and it is in such bad repair that I could not get anything for it if I sold it. I will certainly take care not to give away anything again. One always suffers for being generous."'

'Well?' said the Water-rat, after a long pause.

'Well, that is the end,' said the Linnet.

'But what became of the Miller?' asked the Water-rat.

'Oh! I really don't know,' replied the Linnet; 'and I am sure that I don't care.'

'It is quite evident then that you have no sympathy in your nature,' said the Water-rat.

'I am afraid you don't quite see the moral of the story,' remarked the Linnet.

'The what?' screamed the Water-rat.

'The moral.'

'Do you mean to say that the story has a moral?'

'Certainly,' said the Linnet.

'Well, really,' said the Water-rat, in a very angry manner, 'I think you should have told me that before you began. If you had done so, I certainly would not have listened to you; in fact, I should have said "Pooh", like the critic. However, I can say it now'; so he shouted out 'Pooh' at the top of his voice, gave a whisk with his tail and went back into his hole.

'And how do you like the Water-rat?' asked the Duck, who came paddling up some minutes afterwards. 'He has a great many good points, but for my own part I have a mother's feelings, and I can never look at a confirmed bachelor without the tears coming into my eyes.'

'I am rather afraid that I have annoyed him,' answered the Linnet. 'The fact is, that I told him a story with a moral.'

'Ah! that is always a very dangerous thing to do,' said the Duck.

And I quite agree with her.

THE ADVENTURE OF THE BRUCE-PARTINGTON PLANS

Arthur Conan Doyle

In the third week of November, in the year 1895, a dense yellow fog settled down upon London. From the Monday to the Thursday I doubt whether it was ever possible from our windows in Baker Street to see the loom of the opposite houses. The first day Holmes had spent in cross-indexing his huge book of references. The second and third had been patiently occupied upon a subject which he had recently made his hobby – the music of the Middle Ages. But when, for the fourth time, after pushing back our chairs from breakfast we saw the greasy, heavy brown swirl still drifting past us and condensing in oily drops upon the window-panes, my comrade's impatient and active nature could endure this drab existence no longer. He paced restlessly about our sitting-room in a fever of suppressed energy, biting his nails, tapping the furniture and chafing against inaction.

'Nothing of interest in the paper, Watson?' he said.

I was aware that by anything of interest, Holmes meant anything of criminal interest. There was the news of a revolution, of a possible war and of an impending change of government; but these did not come within the horizon of my companion. I could see nothing recorded in the shape of crime which was not commonplace and futile. Holmes groaned and resumed his restless meanderings.

'The London criminal is certainly a dull fellow,' said he in the querulous voice of the sportsman whose game has failed him. 'Look out this window, Watson. See how the figures loom up, are dimly seen and then blend once more into the cloud-bank. The thief or the murderer could roam London on such a day as the tiger does the jungle, unseen until he pounces, and then evident only to his victim.'

'There have,' said I, 'been numerous petty thefts.'

Holmes snorted his contempt.

'This great and sombre stage is set for something more worthy than that,' said he. 'It is fortunate for this community that I am not a criminal.'

'It is, indeed!' said I heartily.

'Suppose that I were Brooks or Woodhouse, or any of the fifty men who have good reason for taking my life, how long could I survive against my own pursuit? A summons, a bogus appointment, and all would be over. It is well they don't have days of fog in the Latin countries – the countries of assassination. By Jove! here comes something at last to break our dead monotony.'

It was the maid with a telegram. Holmes tore it open and burst out laughing.

'Well, well! What next?' said he. 'Brother Mycroft is coming round.'

'Why not?' I asked.

'Why not? It is as if you met a tram-car coming down a country lane. Mycroft has his rails and he runs on them. His Pall Mall lodgings, the Diogenes Club, Whitehall – that is his cycle. Once, and only once, he has been here. What upheaval can possibly have derailed him?'

'Does he not explain?'

Holmes handed me his brother's telegram.

'Must see you over Cadogan West. Coming at once.'
—MYCROFT.

'Cadogan West? I have heard the name.'

'It recalls nothing to my mind. But that Mycroft should break out in this erratic fashion! A planet might as well leave its orbit. By the way, do you know what Mycroft is?'

I had some vague recollection of an explanation at the time of the Adventure of the Greek Interpreter.

'You told me that he had some small office under the British government.'

Holmes chuckled.

'I did not know you quite so well in those days. One has to be discreet when one talks of high matters of state. You are right in thinking that he is under the British government. You would also be right in a sense if you said that occasionally he *is* the British government.'

'My dear Holmes!'

'I thought I might surprise you. Mycroft draws four hundred and fifty pounds a year, remains a subordinate, has no ambitions of any kind, will receive neither honour nor title, but remains the most indispensable man in the country.'

'But how?'

'Well, his position is unique. He has made it for himself. There has never been anything like it before, nor will be again. He has the tidiest and most orderly brain, with the greatest capacity for storing facts, of any man living. The same great powers which I have turned to the detection of crime he has used for this particular business. The conclusions of every department are passed to him, and he is the central exchange, the clearinghouse, which makes out the balance. All other men are specialists, but his specialism is omniscience. We will suppose that a minister needs information as to a point which involves the Navy, India, Canada and the bimetallic question; he could get his separate advices from various departments upon each, but only Mycroft can focus them all, and say offhand how each factor would affect the other. They began by using him as a short-cut, a convenience; now he has made himself an essential. In that great brain of his everything is pigeon-holed and can be handed out in an instant. Again and again his word has decided the national policy. He lives in it. He thinks of nothing else save when, as an intellectual exercise, he unbends if I call upon him and ask him to advise me on one of my little problems. But Jupiter is descending to-day. What on earth can it mean? Who is Cadogan West, and what is he to Mycroft?'

'I have it,' I cried, and plunged among the litter of papers upon the sofa. 'Yes, yes, here he is, sure enough! Cadogan West was the young man who was found dead on the Underground on Tuesday morning.'

Holmes sat up at attention, his pipe halfway to his lips.

'This must be serious, Watson. A death which has caused my brother to alter his habits can be no ordinary one. What in the world can he have to do with it? The case was featureless as I remember it. The young man had apparently fallen out of the train and killed himself. He had not been robbed, and there was no particular reason to suspect violence. Is that not so?'

'There has been an inquest,' said I, 'and a good many fresh facts have come out. Looked at more closely, I should certainly say that it was a curious case.'

'Judging by its effect upon my brother, I should think it must be a most extraordinary one.' He snuggled down in his armchair. 'Now, Watson, let us have the facts.'

'The man's name was Arthur Cadogan West. He was twenty-seven years of age, unmarried and a clerk at Woolwich Arsenal.'

'Government employ. Behold the link with Brother Mycroft!'

'He left Woolwich suddenly on Monday night. Was last seen by his fiancée, Miss Violet Westbury, whom he left abruptly in the fog about 7:30 that evening. There was no quarrel between them and she can give no motive for his action. The next thing heard of him was when his dead body was discovered by a plate-layer named Mason, just outside Aldgate Station on the Underground system in London.'

'When?'

'The body was found at six on Tuesday morning. It was lying wide of the metals upon the left hand of the track as one goes eastward, at a point close to the station, where the line emerges from the tunnel in which it runs. The head was badly crushed – an injury which might well have been caused by a fall from the train. The body could only have come on the line in that way. Had it been carried down from any neighbouring street, it must have passed the station barriers, where a collector is always standing. This point seems absolutely certain.'

'Very good. The case is definite enough. The man, dead or alive, either fell or was precipitated from a train. So much is clear to me. Continue.'

'The trains which traverse the lines of rail beside which the body was found are those which run from west to east, some being purely Metropolitan, and some from Willesden and outlying junctions. It can be stated for certain that this young man, when he met his death, was travelling in this direction at some late hour of the night, but at what point he entered the train it is impossible to state.'

'His ticket, of course, would show that.'

'There was no ticket in his pockets.'

'No ticket! Dear me, Watson, this is really very singular. According to my experience it is not possible to reach the platform of a Metropolitan train without exhibiting one's ticket. Presumably, then, the young man had one. Was it taken from him in order to conceal the station from which he came? It is possible. Or did he drop it in the carriage? That is also possible. But the point is of curious interest. I understand that there was no sign of robbery?'

'Apparently not. There is a list here of his possessions. His purse contained two pounds fifteen. He had also a cheque-book on the Woolwich branch of the Capital and Counties Bank. Through this his identity was established. There were also two dress-circle tickets for the Woolwich Theatre, dated for that very evening. Also a small packet of technical papers.'

Holmes gave an exclamation of satisfaction.

'There we have it at last, Watson! British government – Woolwich Arsenal – technical papers – Brother Mycroft, the chain is complete. But here he comes, if I am not mistaken, to speak for himself.'

A moment later the tall and portly form of Mycroft Holmes was ushered into the room. Heavily built and massive, there was a suggestion of uncouth physical inertia in the figure, but above this unwieldy frame there was perched a head so masterful in its brow, so alert in its steel-grey, deep-set eyes, so firm in its lips and so subtle in its play of expression, that after the first glance one forgot the gross body and remembered only the dominant mind.

At his heels came our old friend Lestrade, of Scotland Yard – thin and austere. The gravity of both their faces foretold some weighty quest. The detective shook hands without a word. Mycroft Holmes struggled out of his overcoat and subsided into an armchair.

'A most annoying business, Sherlock,' said he. 'I extremely dislike altering my habits, but the powers that be would take no denial. In the present state of Siam it is most awkward that I should be away from the office. But it is a real crisis. I have never seen the Prime Minister so upset. As to the Admiralty – it is buzzing like an overturned bee-hive. Have you read up the case?'

'We have just done so. What were the technical papers?'

'Ah, there's the point! Fortunately, it has not come out. The press would be furious if it did. The papers which this wretched youth had in his pocket were the plans of the Bruce-Partington submarine.'

Mycroft Holmes spoke with a solemnity which showed his sense of the importance of the subject. His brother and I sat expectant.

'Surely you have heard of it? I thought everyone had heard of it.'

'Only as a name.'

'Its importance can hardly be exaggerated. It has been the most jealously guarded of all government secrets. You may take it from me that naval warfare becomes impossible within the radius of a Bruce-Partington's operation. Two years ago a very large sum was smuggled through the Estimates and was expended in acquiring a monopoly of the invention. Every effort has been made to keep the secret. The plans, which are exceedingly intricate, comprising some thirty separate patents, each essential to the working of the whole, are kept in an elaborate safe in a confidential office adjoining the arsenal, with burglar-proof doors and windows. Under no conceivable circumstances were the plans to be taken from the office. If the chief constructor of the Navy desired to consult them, even he was forced to go to the Woolwich office for the purpose. And yet here we find them in the pocket of a dead junior clerk in the heart of London. From an official point of view it's simply awful.'

'But you have recovered them?'

'No, Sherlock, no! That's the pinch. We have not. Ten papers were taken from Woolwich. There were seven in the pocket of Cadogan West. The three most essential are gone – stolen, vanished. You must drop everything, Sherlock. Never mind your usual petty puzzles of the police-court. It's a vital international problem that you have to solve. Why did Cadogan West take the papers, where are the missing ones, how did he die, how came his body where it was found, how can the evil be set right? Find an answer to all these questions, and you will have done good service for your country.'

'Why do you not solve it yourself, Mycroft? You can see as far as I.'

'Possibly, Sherlock. But it is a question of getting details. Give me your details, and from an armchair I will return you an excellent expert opinion. But to run here and run there, to cross-question railway guards and lie on my face with a lens to my eye – it is not my *métier*. No, you are the one man who can clear the matter up. If you have a fancy to see your name in the next honours list—'

My friend smiled and shook his head.

'I play the game for the game's own sake,' said he. 'But the problem certainly presents some points of interest, and I shall be very pleased to look into it. Some more facts, please.'

'I have jotted down the more essential ones upon this sheet of paper, together with a few addresses which you will find of service. The actual official guardian of the papers is the famous government expert, Sir James Walter, whose decorations and sub-titles fill two lines of a book of reference. He has grown grey in the service, is a gentleman, a favoured guest in the most exalted houses and, above all, a man whose patriotism is beyond suspicion. He is one of two who have a key of the safe. I may add that the papers were undoubtedly in the office during working hours on Monday, and that Sir James left for London about three o'clock, taking his key with him. He was at the house of Admiral Sinclair at Barclay Square during the whole of the evening when this incident occurred.'

'Has the fact been verified?'

'Yes; his brother, Colonel Valentine Walter, has testified to his departure from Woolwich, and Admiral Sinclair to his arrival in London; so Sir James is no longer a direct factor in the problem.'

'Who was the other man with a key?'

'The senior clerk and draughtsman, Mr Sidney Johnson. He is a man of forty, married, with five children. He is a silent, morose man, but he has, on the whole, an excellent record in the public service. He is unpopular with his colleagues, but a hard worker. According to his own account, corroborated only by the word of his wife, he was at home the whole of Monday evening after office hours, and his key has never left the watch-chain upon which it hangs.'

'Tell us about Cadogan West.'

'He has been ten years in the service and has done good work. He has the reputation of being hot-headed and imperious, but a straight, honest man. We have nothing against him. He was next Sidney Johnson in the office. His duties brought him into daily, personal contact with the plans. No one else had the handling of them.'

'Who locked up the plans that night?'

'Mr Sidney Johnson, the senior clerk.'

'Well, it is surely perfectly clear who took them away. They are actually found upon the person of this junior clerk, Cadogan West. That seems final, does it not?'

'It does, Sherlock, and yet it leaves so much unexplained. In the first place, why did he take them?'

'I presume they were of value?'

'He could have got several thousands for them very easily.'

'Can you suggest any possible motive for taking the papers to London except to sell them?'

'No, I cannot.'

'Then we must take that as our working hypothesis. Young West took the papers. Now this could only be done by having a false key—'

'Several false keys. He had to open the building and the room.'

'He had, then, several false keys. He took the papers to London to sell the secret, intending, no doubt, to have the plans themselves back in the safe next morning before they were missed. While in London on this treasonable mission he met his end.'

'How?'

'We will suppose that he was travelling back to Woolwich when he was killed and thrown out of the compartment.'

'Aldgate, where the body was found, is considerably past the station London Bridge, which would be his route to Woolwich.'

'Many circumstances could be imagined under which he would pass London Bridge. There was someone in the carriage, for example, with whom he was having an absorbing interview. This interview led to a violent scene in which he lost his life. Possibly he tried to leave the carriage, fell out on the line and so met his end. The other closed the door. There was a thick fog, and nothing could be seen.'

'No better explanation can be given with our present knowledge; and yet consider, Sherlock, how much you leave untouched. We will suppose, for argument's sake, that young Cadogan West *had* determined to convey these papers to London. He would naturally have made an appointment with the foreign agent and kept his evening clear. Instead of that he took two tickets for the theatre, escorted his fiancée halfway there and then suddenly disappeared.'

'A blind,' said Lestrade, who had sat listening with some impatience to the conversation.

'A very singular one. That is objection No. 1. Objection No. 2: We will suppose that he reaches London and sees the foreign agent. He must bring back the papers before morning or the loss will be discovered. He took away ten. Only seven were in his pocket. What had become of the other three? He certainly would not leave them of his own free will. Then, again, where is the price of his treason? One would have expected to find a large sum of money in his pocket.'

'It seems to me perfectly clear,' said Lestrade. 'I have no doubt at all as to what occurred. He took the papers to sell them. He saw the agent. They could not agree as to price. He started home again, but the agent went with him. In the train the agent murdered him, took the more essential papers and threw his body from the carriage. That would account for everything, would it not?'

'Why had he no ticket?'

'The ticket would have shown which station was nearest the agent's house. Therefore he took it from the murdered man's pocket.'

'Good, Lestrade, very good,' said Holmes. 'Your theory holds together. But if this is true, then the case is at an end. On the one hand, the traitor is dead. On the other, the plans of the Bruce-Partington submarine are presumably already on the Continent. What is there for us to do?'

'To act, Sherlock – to act!' cried Mycroft, springing to his feet. 'All my instincts are against this explanation. Use your powers! Go to the scene of the crime! See the people concerned! Leave no stone unturned! In all your career you have never had so great a chance of serving your country.'

'Well, well!' said Holmes, shrugging his shoulders. 'Come, Watson! And you, Lestrade, could you favour us with your company for an hour or two? We will begin our investigation by a visit to Aldgate Station. Good-bye, Mycroft. I shall let you have a report before evening, but I warn you in advance that you have little to expect.'

*

An hour later Holmes, Lestrade and I stood upon the Underground railroad at the point where it emerges from the tunnel immediately before Aldgate Station. A courteous red-faced old gentleman represented the railway company.

'This is where the young man's body lay,' said he, indicating a spot about three feet from the metals. 'It could not have fallen from above, for these, as you see, are all blank walls. Therefore, it could only have come from a train, and that train, so far as we can trace it, must have passed about midnight on Monday.'

'Have the carriages been examined for any sign of violence?'

'There are no such signs, and no ticket has been found.'

'No record of a door being found open?'

'None.'

'We have had some fresh evidence this morning,' said Lestrade. 'A passenger who passed Aldgate in an ordinary Metropolitan train about 11:40 on Monday night declares that he heard a heavy thud, as of a body striking the line, just before the train reached the station. There was dense fog, however, and nothing could be seen. He made no report of it at the time. Why, whatever is the matter with Mr Holmes?'

My friend was standing with an expression of strained intensity upon his face, staring at the railway metals where they curved out of the tunnel. Aldgate is a junction, and there was a network of points. On these his eager, questioning eyes were fixed, and I saw on his keen, alert face that tightening of the lips, that quiver of the nostrils and concentration of the heavy, tufted brows which I knew so well.

'Points,' he muttered; 'the points.'

'What of it? What do you mean?'

'I suppose there are no great number of points on a system such as this?'

'No; they are very few.'

'And a curve, too. Points, and a curve. By Jove! if it were only so.'

'What is it, Mr Holmes? Have you a clue?'

'An idea – an indication, no more. But the case certainly grows in interest. Unique, perfectly unique, and yet why not? I do not see any indications of bleeding on the line.'

'There were hardly any.'

'But I understand that there was a considerable wound.'

'The bone was crushed, but there was no great external injury.'

'And yet one would have expected some bleeding. Would it be possible for me to inspect the train which contained the passenger who heard the thud of a fall in the fog?'

'I fear not, Mr Holmes. The train has been broken up before now, and the carriages redistributed.'

'I can assure you, Mr Holmes,' said Lestrade, 'that every carriage has been carefully examined. I saw to it myself.'

It was one of my friend's most obvious weaknesses that he was impatient with less alert intelligences than his own.

'Very likely,' said he, turning away. 'As it happens, it was not the carriages which I desired to examine. Watson, we have done all we can here. We need not trouble you any further, Mr Lestrade. I think our investigations must now carry us to Woolwich.'

At London Bridge, Holmes wrote a telegram to his brother, which he handed to me before dispatching it. It ran thus:

See some light in the darkness, but it may possibly flicker out. Meanwhile, please send by messenger, to await return at Baker Street, a complete list of all foreign spies or international agents known to be in England, with full address.
—SHERLOCK.

'That should be helpful, Watson,' he remarked as we took our seats in the Woolwich train. 'We certainly owe Brother Mycroft a debt for having introduced us to what promises to be a really very remarkable case.'

His eager face still wore that expression of intense and high-strung energy, which showed me that some novel and suggestive circumstance had opened up a stimulating line of thought. See the foxhound with hanging ears and drooping tail as it lolls about the kennels, and compare it with the same hound as, with gleaming eyes and straining muscles, it runs upon a breast-high scent – such was the change in Holmes since the morning. He was a different man from the limp and lounging figure in the mouse-coloured dressing-gown who had prowled so restlessly only a few hours before round the fog-girt room.

'There is material here. There is scope,' said he. 'I am dull indeed not to have understood its possibilities.'

'Even now they are dark to me.'

'The end is dark to me also, but I have hold of one idea which may lead us far. The man met his death elsewhere, and his body was on the *roof* of a carriage.'

'On the roof!'

'Remarkable, is it not? But consider the facts. Is it a coincidence that it is found at the very point where the train pitches and sways as it comes round on the points? Is not that the place where an object upon the roof might be expected to fall off? The points would affect no object inside the train. Either the body fell from the roof, or a very curious coincidence has occurred. But now consider the question of the blood. Of course, there was no bleeding on the line if the body had bled elsewhere. Each fact is suggestive in itself. Together they have a cumulative force.'

'And the ticket, too!' I cried.

'Exactly. We could not explain the absence of a ticket. This would explain it. Everything fits together.'

'But suppose it were so, we are still as far as ever from unravelling the mystery of his death. Indeed, it becomes not simpler but stranger.'

'Perhaps,' said Holmes, thoughtfully, 'perhaps.' He relapsed into a silent reverie, which lasted until the slow train drew up at last in Woolwich Station. There he called a cab and drew Mycroft's paper from his pocket.

'We have quite a little round of afternoon calls to make,' said he. 'I think that Sir James Walter claims our first attention.'

The house of the famous official was a fine villa with green lawns stretching down to the Thames. As we reached it the fog was lifting, and a thin, watery sunshine was breaking through. A butler answered our ring.

'Sir James, sir!' said he with solemn face. 'Sir James died this morning.'

'Good heavens!' cried Holmes in amazement. 'How did he die?'

'Perhaps you would care to step in, sir, and see his brother, Colonel Valentine?'

'Yes, we had best do so.'

We were ushered into a dim-lit drawing-room, where an instant later we were joined by a very tall, handsome, light-bearded man of fifty, the younger brother of the dead scientist. His wild eyes, stained cheeks and unkempt hair all spoke of the sudden blow which had fallen upon the household. He was hardly articulate as he spoke of it.

'It was this horrible scandal,' said he. 'My brother, Sir James, was a man of very sensitive honour, and he could not survive such an affair. It broke his heart. He was always so proud of the efficiency of his department, and this was a crushing blow.'

'We had hoped that he might have given us some indications which would have helped us to clear the matter up.'

'I assure you that it was all a mystery to him as it is to you and to all of us. He had already put all his knowledge at the disposal of the police. Naturally he had no doubt that Cadogan West was guilty. But all the rest was inconceivable.'

'You cannot throw any new light upon the affair?'

'I know nothing myself save what I have read or heard. I have no desire to be discourteous, but you can understand, Mr Holmes, that we are much disturbed at present, and I must ask you to hasten this interview to an end.'

'This is indeed an unexpected development,' said my friend when we had regained the cab. 'I wonder if the death was natural, or whether the poor old fellow killed himself! If the latter, may it be taken as some sign of self-reproach for duty neglected? We must leave that question to the future. Now we shall turn to the Cadogan Wests.'

A small but well-kept house in the outskirts of the town sheltered the bereaved mother. The old lady was too dazed with grief to be of any use to us, but at her side was a white-faced young lady, who introduced herself as Miss Violet Westbury, the fiancée of the dead man, and the last to see him upon that fatal night.

'I cannot explain it, Mr Holmes,' she said. 'I have not shut an eye since the tragedy, thinking, thinking, thinking, night and day, what the true meaning of it can be. Arthur was the most single-minded, chivalrous, patriotic man upon earth. He would have cut his right hand off before he would sell a State secret confided to his keeping. It is absurd, impossible, preposterous to anyone who knew him.'

'But the facts, Miss Westbury?'

'Yes, yes; I admit I cannot explain them.'

'Was he in any want of money?'

'No; his needs were very simple and his salary ample. He had saved a few hundreds, and we were to marry at the New Year.'

'No signs of any mental excitement? Come, Miss Westbury, be absolutely frank with us.'

The quick eye of my companion had noted some change in her manner. She coloured and hesitated.

'Yes,' she said at last, 'I had a feeling that there was something on his mind.'

'For long?'

'Only for the last week or so. He was thoughtful and worried. Once I pressed him about it. He admitted that there was something, and that it was concerned with his official life. "It is too serious for me to speak about, even to you," said he. I could get nothing more.'

Holmes looked grave.

'Go on, Miss Westbury. Even if it seems to tell against him, go on. We cannot say what it may lead to.'

'Indeed, I have nothing more to tell. Once or twice it seemed to me that he was on the point of telling me something. He spoke one evening of the importance of the secret, and I have some recollection that he said that no doubt foreign spies would pay a great deal to have it.'

My friend's face grew graver still.

'Anything else?'

'He said that we were slack about such matters – that it would be easy for a traitor to get the plans.'

'Was it only recently that he made such remarks?'

'Yes, quite recently.'

'Now tell us of that last evening.'

'We were to go to the theatre. The fog was so thick that a cab was useless. We walked, and our way took us close to the office. Suddenly he darted away into the fog.'

'Without a word?'

'He gave an exclamation; that was all. I waited but he never returned. Then I walked home. Next morning, after the office opened, they came to inquire. About twelve o'clock we heard the terrible news. Oh, Mr Holmes, if you could only, only save his honour! It was so much to him.'

Holmes shook his head sadly.

'Come, Watson,' said he, 'our ways lie elsewhere. Our next station must be the office from which the papers were taken.

'It was black enough before against this young man, but our inquiries make it blacker,' he remarked as the cab lumbered off. 'His coming marriage gives a motive for the crime. He naturally wanted money. The idea was in his head, since he spoke about it. He nearly made the girl an accomplice in the treason by telling her his plans. It is all very bad.'

'But surely, Holmes, character goes for something? Then, again, why should he leave the girl in the street and dart away to commit a felony?'

'Exactly! There are certainly objections. But it is a formidable case which they have to meet.'

Mr Sidney Johnson, the senior clerk, met us at the office and received us with that respect which my companion's card always commanded. He was a thin, gruff, bespectacled man of middle age, his cheeks haggard, and his hands twitching from the nervous strain to which he had been subjected.

'It is bad, Mr Holmes, very bad! Have you heard of the death of the chief?'

'We have just come from his house.'

'The place is disorganized. The chief dead, Cadogan West dead, our papers stolen. And yet, when we closed our door on Monday evening, we were as efficient an office as any in the government service. Good God, it's dreadful to think of! That West, of all men, should have done such a thing!'

'You are sure of his guilt, then?'

'I can see no other way out of it. And yet I would have trusted him as I trust myself.'

'At what hour was the office closed on Monday?'

'At five.'

'Did you close it?'

'I am always the last man out.'

'Where were the plans?'

'In that safe. I put them there myself.'

'Is there no watchman to the building?'

'There is, but he has other departments to look after as well. He is an old soldier and a most trustworthy man. He saw nothing that evening. Of course the fog was very thick.'

'Suppose that Cadogan West wished to make his way into the building after hours; he would need three keys, would he not, before he could reach the papers?'

'Yes, he would. The key of the outer door, the key of the office and the key of the safe.'

'Only Sir James Walter and you had those keys?'

'I had no keys of the doors – only of the safe.'

'Was Sir James a man who was orderly in his habits?'

'Yes, I think he was. I know that so far as those three keys are concerned he kept them on the same ring. I have often seen them there.'

'And that ring went with him to London?'

'He said so.'

'And your key never left your possession?'

'Never.'

'Then West, if he is the culprit, must have had a duplicate. And yet none was found upon his body. One other point: if a clerk in this office desired to sell the plans, would it not be simpler to copy the plans for himself than to take the originals, as was actually done?'

'It would take considerable technical knowledge to copy the plans in an effective way.'

'But I suppose either Sir James, or you, or West has that technical knowledge?'

'No doubt we had, but I beg you won't try to drag me into the matter, Mr Holmes. What is the use of our speculating in this way when the original plans were actually found on West?'

'Well, it is certainly singular that he should run the risk of taking originals if he could safely have taken copies, which would have equally served his turn.'

'Singular, no doubt – and yet he did so.'

'Every inquiry in this case reveals something inexplicable. Now there are three papers still missing. They are, as I understand, the vital ones.'

'Yes, that is so.'

'Do you mean to say that anyone holding these three papers, and without the seven others, could construct a Bruce-Partington submarine?'

'I reported to that effect to the Admiralty. But to-day I have been over the drawings again, and I am not so sure of it. The double valves with the automatic self-adjusting slots are drawn in one of the papers which have been returned. Until the foreigners had invented that for themselves they could not make the boat. Of course they might soon get over the difficulty.'

'But the three missing drawings are the most important?'

'Undoubtedly.'

'I think, with your permission, I will now take a stroll round the premises. I do not recall any other question which I desired to ask.'

He examined the lock of the safe, the door of the room and finally the iron shutters of the window. It was only when we were on the lawn outside that his interest was strongly excited. There was a laurel bush outside the window, and several of the branches bore signs of having been twisted or snapped. He examined them carefully with his lens, and then some dim and vague marks upon the earth beneath. Finally he asked the chief clerk to close the iron shutters, and he pointed out to me that they hardly met in the centre, and that it would be possible for anyone outside to see what was going on within the room.

'The indications are ruined by three days' delay. They may mean something or nothing. Well, Watson, I do not think that Woolwich can help us further. It is a small crop which we have gathered. Let us see if we can do better in London.'

Yet we added one more sheaf to our harvest before we left Woolwich Station. The clerk in the ticket office was able to say with confidence that he saw Cadogan West – whom he knew well by sight – upon the Monday night, and that he went to London by the 8:15 to London Bridge. He was alone and took a single third-class ticket. The clerk was struck at the time by his excited and nervous manner. So shaky was he that he could hardly pick up his change, and the clerk had helped him with it. A reference to the timetable showed that the 8:15 was the first train which it was possible for West to take after he had left the lady about 7:30.

'Let us reconstruct, Watson,' said Holmes after half an hour of silence. 'I am not aware that in all our joint researches we have ever had a case which was more difficult to get at. Every fresh advance which we make only reveals a fresh ridge beyond. And yet we have surely made some appreciable progress.

'The effect of our inquiries at Woolwich has in the main been against young Cadogan West; but the indications at the window would lend themselves to a more favourable hypothesis. Let us suppose, for example, that he had been approached by some foreign agent. It might have been done under such pledges as would have prevented him from speaking of it, and yet would have affected his thoughts in the direction indicated by his remarks to his fiancée. Very good. We will now suppose that as he went to the theatre with the young lady he suddenly, in the fog, caught a glimpse of this same agent going in the direction of the office. He was an impetuous man, quick in his decisions. Everything gave way to his duty. He followed the man, reached the window, saw the abstraction of the documents and pursued the thief. In this way we get over the objection that no one would take originals when he could make copies. This outsider had to take originals. So far it holds together.'

'What is the next step?'

'Then we come into difficulties. One would imagine that under such circumstances the first act of young Cadogan West would be to seize the villain and raise the alarm. Why did he not do so? Could it have been an official superior who took the papers? That would explain West's conduct. Or could the chief have given West the slip in the fog, and West started at once to London to head him off from his own rooms, presuming that he knew where the rooms were? The call must have been very pressing, since he left his girl standing in the fog and made no effort to communicate with her. Our scent runs cold here, and there is a vast gap between either hypothesis and the laying of West's body, with seven papers in his pocket, on the roof of a Metropolitan train. My instinct now is to work from the other end. If Mycroft has given us the list of addresses we may be able to pick our man and follow two tracks instead of one.'

Surely enough, a note awaited us at Baker Street. A government messenger had brought it post-haste. Holmes glanced at it and threw it over to me.

There are numerous small fry, but few who would handle so big an affair. The only men worth considering are Adolph Mayer, of 13, Great George Street, Westminster; Louis La Rothière, of Campden Mansions, Notting Hill; and Hugo Oberstein, 13, Caulfield Gardens, Kensington. The latter was known to be in town on Monday and is now reported as having left. Glad to hear you have seen some light. The Cabinet awaits your final report with the utmost anxiety. Urgent representations have arrived from the very highest quarter. The whole force of the State is at your back if you should need it.—MYCROFT.

'I'm afraid,' said Holmes, smiling, 'that all the Queen's horses and all the Queen's men cannot avail in this matter.' He had spread out his big map of London and leaned eagerly over it. 'Well, well,' said he presently with an exclamation of satisfaction, 'things are turning a little in our direction at last. Why, Watson, I do honestly believe that we are going to pull it off, after all.' He slapped me on the shoulder with a sudden burst of hilarity. 'I am going out now. It is only a reconnaissance. I will do nothing serious without my trusted comrade and biographer at my elbow. Do you stay here, and the odds are that you will see me again in an hour or two. If time hangs heavy get foolscap and a pen, and begin your narrative of how we saved the State.'

I felt some reflection of his elation in my own mind, for I knew well that he would not depart so far from his usual austerity of demeanour unless there was good cause for exultation. All the long November evening I waited, filled with impatience for his return. At last, shortly after nine o'clock, there arrived a messenger with a note:

Am dining at Goldini's Restaurant, Gloucester Road, Kensington.

Please come at once and join me there. Bring with you a jemmy, a dark lantern, a chisel and a revolver.—S H

It was a nice equipment for a respectable citizen to carry through the dim, fog-draped streets. I stowed them all discreetly away in my overcoat and drove straight to the address given. There sat my friend at a little round table near the door of the garish Italian restaurant.

'Have you had something to eat? Then join me in a coffee and curaçao. Try one of the proprietor's cigars. They are less poisonous than one would expect. Have you the tools?'

'They are here, in my overcoat.'

'Excellent. Let me give you a short sketch of what I have done, with some indication of what we are about to do. Now it must be evident to you, Watson, that this young man's body was *placed* on the roof of the train. That was clear from the instant that I determined the fact that it was from the roof, and not from a carriage, that he had fallen.'

'Could it not have been dropped from a bridge?'

'I should say it was impossible. If you examine the roofs you will find that they are slightly rounded, and there is no railing round them. Therefore, we can say for certain that young Cadogan West was placed on it.'

'How could he be placed there?'

'That was the question which we had to answer. There is only one possible way. You are aware that the Underground runs clear of tunnels at some points in the West End. I had a vague memory that as I have travelled by it I have occasionally seen windows just above my head. Now, suppose that a train halted under such a window, would there be any difficulty in laying a body upon the roof?'

'It seems most improbable.'

'We must fall back upon the old axiom that when all other

contingencies fail, whatever remains, however improbable, must be the truth. Here all other contingencies have failed. When I found that the leading international agent, who had just left London, lived in a row of houses which abutted upon the Underground, I was so pleased that you were a little astonished at my sudden frivolity.'

'Oh, that was it, was it?'

'Yes, that was it. Mr Hugo Oberstein, of 13, Caulfield Gardens, had become my objective. I began my operations at Gloucester Road Station, where a very helpful official walked with me along the track and allowed me to satisfy myself not only that the backstair windows of Caulfield Gardens open on the line but the even more essential fact that, owing to the intersection of one of the larger railways, the Underground trains are frequently held motionless for some minutes at that very spot.'

'Splendid, Holmes! You have got it!'

'So far – so far, Watson. We advance, but the goal is afar. Well, having seen the back of Caulfield Gardens, I visited the front and satisfied myself that the bird was indeed flown. It is a considerable house, unfurnished, so far as I could judge, in the upper rooms. Oberstein lived there with a single valet, who was probably a confederate entirely in his confidence. We must bear in mind that Oberstein has gone to the Continent to dispose of his booty, but not with any idea of flight; for he had no reason to fear a warrant, and the idea of an amateur domiciliary visit would certainly never occur to him. Yet that is precisely what we are about to make.'

'Could we not get a warrant and legalize it?'

'Hardly on the evidence.'

'What can we hope to do?'

'We cannot tell what correspondence may be there.'

'I don't like it, Holmes.'

'My dear fellow, you shall keep watch in the street. I'll do the criminal part. It's not a time to stick at trifles. Think of Mycroft's note, of the Admiralty, the Cabinet, the exalted person who waits for news. We are bound to go.'

My answer was to rise from the table.

'You are right, Holmes. We are bound to go.'

He sprang up and shook me by the hand.

'I knew you would not shrink at the last,' said he, and for a moment I saw something in his eyes which was nearer to tenderness than I had ever seen. The next instant he was his masterful, practical self once more.

'It is nearly half a mile, but there is no hurry. Let us walk,' said he. 'Don't drop the instruments, I beg. Your arrest as a suspicious character would be a most unfortunate complication.'

Caulfield Gardens was one of those lines of flat-faced, pillared and porticoed houses which are so prominent a product of the middle Victorian epoch in the West End of London. Next door there appeared to be a children's party, for the merry buzz of young voices and the clatter of a piano resounded through the night. The fog still hung about and screened us with its friendly shade. Holmes had lit his lantern and flashed it upon the massive door.

'This is a serious proposition,' said he. 'It is certainly bolted as well as locked. We would do better in the area. There is an excellent archway down yonder in case a too zealous policeman should intrude. Give me a hand, Watson, and I'll do the same for you.'

A minute later we were both in the area. Hardly had we reached the dark shadows before the step of the policeman was heard in the fog above. As its soft rhythm died away, Holmes set to work upon the lower door. I saw him stoop and strain until with a sharp crash it flew open. We sprang through into the dark passage, closing the area door behind us. Holmes led the way up the curving, uncarpeted stair. His little fan of yellow light shone upon a low window.

'Here we are, Watson – this must be the one.' He threw it open, and as he did so there was a low, harsh murmur, growing steadily into a loud roar as a train dashed past us in the darkness. Holmes swept his light along the window-sill. It was thickly coated with soot from the passing engines, but the black surface was blurred and rubbed in places.

'You can see where they rested the body. Halloa, Watson! what is this? There can be no doubt that it is a blood mark.' He was pointing to faint discolorations along the woodwork of the window. 'Here it is on the stone of the stair also. The demonstration is complete. Let us stay here until a train stops.'

We had not long to wait. The very next train roared from the tunnel as before, but slowed in the open, and then, with a creaking of brakes, pulled up immediately beneath us. It was not four feet from the window-ledge to the roof of the carriages. Holmes softly closed the window.

'So far we are justified,' said he. 'What do you think of it, Watson?'

'A masterpiece. You have never risen to a greater height.'

'I cannot agree with you there. From the moment that I conceived the idea of the body being upon the roof, which surely was not a very abstruse one, all the rest was inevitable. If it were not for the grave interests involved the affair up to this point would be insignificant. Our difficulties are still before us. But perhaps we may find something here which may help us.'

We had ascended the kitchen stair and entered the suite of rooms upon the first floor. One was a dining-room, severely furnished and containing nothing of interest. A second was a bedroom, which also drew blank. The remaining room appeared more promising, and my companion settled down to a systematic examination. It was littered with books and papers, and was evidently used as a study. Swiftly and methodically Holmes turned over the contents of drawer after drawer and cupboard after cupboard, but no gleam of success came to brighten his austere face. At the end of an hour he was no further than when he started.

'The cunning dog has covered his tracks,' said he. 'He has left nothing to incriminate him. His dangerous correspondence has been destroyed or removed. This is our last chance.'

It was a small tin cash-box which stood upon the writing-desk. Holmes pried it open with his chisel. Several rolls of paper were within, covered with figures and calculations, without any note to show to what they referred. The recurring words, 'water pressure' and 'pressure to the square inch' suggested some possible relation to a submarine. Holmes tossed them all impatiently aside. There only remained an envelope with some small newspaper slips inside it. He shook them out on the table, and at once I saw by his eager face that his hopes had been raised.

'What's this, Watson? Eh? What's this? Record of a series of messages in the advertisements of a paper. *Daily Telegraph* agony column by the print and paper. Right-hand top corner of a page. No dates – but messages arrange themselves. This must be the first:

Hoped to hear sooner. Terms agreed to. Write fully to address given on card.—Pierrot.

'Next comes:

Too complex for description. Must have full report. Stuff awaits you when goods delivered.—Pierrot.

'Then comes:

Matter presses. Must withdraw offer unless contract completed. Make appointment by letter. Will confirm by advertisement.—Pierrot.

'Finally:

Monday night after nine. Two taps. Only ourselves. Do not be so suspicious. Payment in hard cash when goods delivered.—Pierrot.

'A fairly complete record, Watson! If we could only get at the man at the other end!' He sat lost in thought, tapping his fingers on the table. Finally he sprang to his feet.

'Well, perhaps it won't be so difficult, after all. There is nothing more to be done here, Watson. I think we might drive round to the offices of the *Daily Telegraph*, and so bring a good day's work to a conclusion.'

Mycroft Holmes and Lestrade had come round by appointment after breakfast next day and Sherlock Holmes had recounted to them our proceedings of the day before. The professional shook his head over our confessed burglary.

'We can't do these things in the force, Mr Holmes,' said he. 'No wonder you get results that are beyond us. But some of these days you'll go too far, and you'll find yourself and your friend in trouble.'

'For England, home and beauty – eh, Watson? Martyrs on the altar of our country. But what do you think of it, Mycroft?'

'Excellent, Sherlock! Admirable! But what use will you make of it?'

Holmes picked up the *Daily Telegraph* which lay upon the table.

'Have you seen Pierrot's advertisement to-day?'

'What? Another one?'

'Yes, here it is:

To-night. Same hour. Same place. Two taps. Most vitally important. Your own safety at stake.—Pierrot.

'By George!' cried Lestrade. 'If he answers that we've got him!'

'That was my idea when I put it in. I think if you could both make it convenient to come with us about eight o'clock to Caulfield Gardens we might possibly get a little nearer to a solution.'

One of the most remarkable characteristics of Sherlock Holmes was his power of throwing his brain out of action and switching all his thoughts on to lighter things whenever he had convinced himself that he could no longer work to advantage. I remember that during the whole of that memorable day he lost himself in a monograph which he had undertaken upon the Polyphonic Motets of Lassus. For my own part I had none of this power of detachment, and the day, in consequence, appeared to be interminable. The great national importance of the issue, the suspense in high quarters, the direct nature of the experiment which we were trying – all combined to work upon my nerve. It was a relief to me when at last, after a light dinner, we set out upon our expedition. Lestrade and Mycroft met us by appointment at the outside of Gloucester Road Station. The area door of Oberstein's house had been left open the night before, and it was necessary for me, as Mycroft Holmes absolutely and indignantly declined to climb the railings, to pass in and open the hall door. By nine o'clock we were all seated in the study, waiting patiently for our man.

An hour passed and yet another. When eleven struck, the measured beat of the great church clock seemed to sound the dirge of our hopes. Lestrade and Mycroft were fidgeting in their seats and looking twice a minute at their watches. Holmes sat silent and composed, his eyelids half shut, but every sense on the alert. He raised his head with a sudden jerk.

'He is coming,' said he.

There had been a furtive step past the door. Now it returned. We heard a shuffling sound outside, and then two sharp taps with the knocker. Holmes rose, motioning us to remain seated. The gas in the hall was a mere point of light. He opened the outer door, and then as a dark figure slipped past him he closed and fastened it. 'This way!' we heard him say, and a moment later our man stood before us. Holmes had followed him closely, and as the man turned with a cry of surprise and alarm he caught him by the collar and threw him back into the room. Before our prisoner had recovered his balance the door was shut and Holmes standing with his back against it. The man glared round him, staggered and fell senseless upon the floor. With the shock, his broad-brimmed hat flew from his head, his cravat slipped down from his lips and there were the long light beard and the soft, handsome delicate features of Colonel Valentine Walter.

Holmes gave a whistle of surprise.

'You can write me down an ass this time, Watson,' said he. 'This was not the bird that I was looking for.'

'Who is he?' asked Mycroft eagerly.

'The younger brother of the late Sir James Walter, the head of the Submarine Department. Yes, yes; I see the fall of the cards. He is coming to. I think that you had best leave his examination to me.'

We had carried the prostrate body to the sofa. Now our prisoner sat up, looked round him with a horror-stricken face, and passed his hand over his forehead, like one who cannot believe his own senses.

'What is this?' he asked. 'I came here to visit Mr Oberstein.'

'Everything is known, Colonel Walter,' said Holmes. 'How an English gentleman could behave in such a manner is beyond my comprehension. But your whole correspondence and relations with Oberstein are within our knowledge. So also are the circumstances connected with the death of young Cadogan West. Let me advise you to gain at least the small credit for repentance and confession, since there are still some details which we can only learn from your lips.'

The man groaned and sank his face in his hands. We waited, but he was silent.

'I can assure you,' said Holmes, 'that every essential is already known. We know that you were pressed for money; that you took an impress of the keys which your brother held; and that you entered into a correspondence with Oberstein, who answered your letters through the advertisement columns of the *Daily Telegraph*. We are aware that you went down to the office in the fog on Monday night, but that you were seen and followed by young Cadogan West, who had probably some previous reason to suspect you. He saw your theft, but could not give the alarm, as it was just possible that you were taking the papers to your brother in London. Leaving all his private concerns, like the good citizen that he was, he followed you closely in the fog and kept at your heels until you reached this very house. There he intervened, and then it was, Colonel Walter, that to treason you added the more terrible crime of murder.'

'I did not! I did not! Before God I swear that I did not!' cried our wretched prisoner.

'Tell us, then, how Cadogan West met his end before you laid him upon the roof of a railway carriage.'

'I will. I swear to you that I will. I did the rest. I confess it. It was just as you say. A Stock Exchange debt had to be paid. I needed the money badly. Oberstein offered me five thousand. It was to save myself from ruin. But as to murder, I am as innocent as you.'

'What happened, then?'

'He had his suspicions before, and he followed me as you describe. I never knew it until I was at the very door. It was thick fog, and one could not see three yards. I had given two taps and Oberstein had come to the door. The young man rushed up and demanded to know what we were about to do with the papers. Oberstein had a short life-preserver. He always carried it with him. As West forced his way after us into the house Oberstein struck him on the head. The blow was a fatal one. He was dead within five minutes. There he lay in the hall, and we were at our wits' end what to do. Then Oberstein had this idea about the trains which halted under his back window. But first he examined the papers which I had brought. He said that three of them were essential, and that he must keep them. "You cannot keep them," said I. "There will be a dreadful row at Woolwich if they are not returned." "I must keep them," said he, "for they are so technical that it is impossible in the time to make copies." "Then they must all go back together to-night," said I. He thought for a little, and then he cried out that he had it. "Three I will keep," said he. "The others we will stuff into the pocket of this young man. When he is found the whole business will assuredly be put to his account." I could see no other way out of it, so we did as he suggested. We waited half an hour at the window before a train stopped. It was so thick that nothing could be seen, and we had no difficulty in lowering West's body on to the train. That was the end of the matter so far as I was concerned.'

'And your brother?'

'He said nothing, but he had caught me once with his keys, and I think that he suspected. I read in his eyes that he suspected. As you know, he never held up his head again.'

There was silence in the room. It was broken by Mycroft Holmes.

'Can you not make reparation? It would ease your conscience, and possibly your punishment.'

'What reparation can I make?'

'Where is Oberstein with the papers?'

'I do not know.'

'Did he give you no address?'

'He said that letters to the Hôtel du Louvre, Paris, would eventually reach him.'

'Then reparation is still within your power,' said Sherlock Holmes.

'I will do anything I can. I owe this fellow no particular good-will. He has been my ruin and my downfall.'

'Here are paper and pen. Sit at this desk and write to my dictation. Direct the envelope to the address given. That is right. Now the letter:

'"Dear Sir:

'"With regard to our transaction, you will no doubt have observed by now that one essential detail is missing. I have a tracing which will make it complete. This has involved me in extra trouble, however, and I must ask you for a further advance of five hundred pounds. I will not trust it to the post, nor will I take anything but gold or notes. I would come to you abroad, but it would excite remark if I left the country at present. Therefore I shall expect to meet you in the smoking-room of the Charing Cross Hotel at noon on Saturday. Remember that only English notes, or gold, will be taken."

'That will do very well. I shall be very much surprised if it does not fetch our man.'

*

And it did! It is a matter of history – that secret history of a nation which is often so much more intimate and interesting than its public chronicles – that Oberstein, eager to complete the coup of his lifetime, came to the lure and was safely engulfed for fifteen years in a British prison. In his trunk were found the invaluable Bruce-Partington plans, which he had put up for auction in all the naval centres of Europe.

Colonel Walter died in prison towards the end of the second year of his sentence. As to Holmes, he returned refreshed to his monograph upon the Polyphonic Motets of Lassus, which has since been printed for private circulation, and is said by experts to be the last word upon the subject. Some weeks afterwards I learned incidentally that my friend spent a day at Windsor, whence he returned with a remarkably fine emerald tie-pin. When I asked him if he had bought it, he answered that it was a present from a certain gracious lady in whose interests he had once been fortunate enough to carry out a small commission. He said no more; but I fancy that I could guess at that lady's august name, and I have little doubt that the emerald pin will forever recall to my friend's memory the adventure of the Bruce-Partington plans.

THE GIANT BUILDER

Abbie Farwell Brown

Ages and ages ago, when the world was first made, the gods decided to build a beautiful city high above the heavens, the most glorious and wonderful city that ever was known. Asgard was to be its name, and it was to stand on Ida Plain under the shade of Yggdrasil, the great tree whose roots were underneath the earth.

First of all they built a house with a silver roof, where there were seats for all the twelve chiefs. In the midst, and high above the rest, was the wonder-throne of Odin the All-Father, whence he could see everything that happened in the sky or on the earth or in the sea. Next they made a fair house for Queen Frigg and her lovely daughters. Then they built a smithy, with its great hammers, tongs, anvils and bellows, where the gods could work at their favourite trade, the making of beautiful things out of gold; which they did so well that folk name that time the Golden Age. Afterwards, as they had more leisure, they built separate houses for all the Æsir, each more beautiful than the preceding, for of course they were continually growing more skilful. They saved Father Odin's palace until the last, for they meant this to be the largest and the most splendid of all.

Gladsheim, the home of joy, was the name of Odin's house, and it was built all of gold, set in the midst of a wood whereof the trees had leaves of ruddy gold – like an autumn-gilded forest. For the safety of All-Father it was surrounded by a roaring river and by a high picket fence; and there was a great courtyard within.

The glory of Gladsheim was its wondrous hall, radiant with gold, the most lovely room that time has ever seen. Valhalla, the Hall of Heroes, was the name of it, and it was roofed with the mighty shields of warriors. The ceiling was made of interlacing spears, and there was a portal at the west end before which hung a great grey wolf, while over him a fierce eagle hovered. The hall was so huge that it had 540 gates, through each of which 800 men could march abreast. Indeed, there needed to be room, for this was the hall where every morning Odin received all the brave warriors who had died in battle on the earth below; and there were many heroes in those days.

This was the reward which the gods gave to courage. When a hero had gloriously lost his life, the Valkyries, the nine warrior daughters of Odin, brought his body up to Valhalla on their white horses that gallop the clouds. There they lived forever after in happiness, enjoying the things that they had most loved upon earth. Every morning they armed themselves and went out to fight with one another in the great courtyard. It was a wondrous game, wondrously played. No matter how often a hero was killed, he became alive again in time to return perfectly well to Valhalla, where he ate a delicious breakfast with the Æsir; while the beautiful Valkyries who had first brought him thither waited at table and poured the blessed mead, which only the immortal taste. A happy life it was for the heroes, and a happy life for all who dwelt in Asgard; for this was before trouble had come among the gods, following the mischief of Loki.

This is how the trouble began. From the beginning of time, the giants had been unfriendly to the Æsir, because the giants were older and huger and more wicked; besides, they were jealous because the good Æsir were fast gaining more wisdom and power than the giants had ever known. It was the Æsir who set the fair brother and sister, Sun and Moon, in the sky to give light to men; and it was they also who made the jewelled stars out of sparks from the place of fire. The giants hated the Æsir, and tried all in their power to injure them and the men of the earth below, whom the Æsir loved and cared for. The gods had already built a wall around Midgard, the world of men, to keep the giants out; built it of the bushy eyebrows of Ymir, the oldest and hugest of giants. Between Asgard and the giants flowed Ifing, the great river on which ice never formed, and which the gods crossed on the rainbow bridge. But this was not protection enough. Their beautiful new city needed a fortress.

So the word went forth in Asgard – 'We must build us a fortress against the giants; the hugest, strongest, finest fortress that ever was built.'

Now one day, soon after they had announced this decision, there came a mighty man stalking up the rainbow bridge that led to Asgard city.

'Who goes there!' cried Heimdal the watchman, whose eyes were so keen that he could see for a hundred miles around, and whose ears were so sharp that he could hear the grass growing in the meadow and the wool on the backs of the sheep. 'Who goes there! No one can enter Asgard if I say no.'

'I am a builder,' said the stranger, who was a huge fellow with sleeves rolled up to show the iron muscles of his arms. 'I am a builder of strong towers, and I have heard that the folk of Asgard need one to help them raise a fair fortress in their city.'

Heimdal looked at the stranger narrowly, for there was that about him which his sharp eyes did not like. But he made no answer, only blew on his golden horn, which was so loud that it sounded through all the world. At this signal all the Æsir came running to the rainbow bridge, from wherever they happened to be, to find out who was coming to Asgard. For it was Heimdal's duty ever to warn them of the approach of the unknown.

'This fellow says he is a builder,' quoth Heimdal. 'And he would fain build us a fortress in the city.'

'Ay, that I would,' nodded the stranger. 'Look at my iron arm; look at my broad back; look at my shoulders. Am I not the workman you need?'

'Truly, he is a mighty figure,' vowed Odin, looking at him approvingly. 'How long will it take you alone to build our fortress? We can allow but one stranger at a time within our city, for safety's sake.'

'In three half-years,' replied the stranger, 'I will undertake to build for you a castle so strong that not even the giants, should they swarm hither over Midgard – not even they could enter without your leave.'

'Aha!' cried Father Odin, well pleased at this offer. 'And what reward do you ask, friend, for help so timely?'

The stranger hummed and hawed and pulled his long beard while he thought. Then he spoke suddenly, as if the idea had just come into his mind. 'I will name my price, friends,' he said; 'a small price for so great a deed. I ask you to give me Freia for my wife, and those two sparkling jewels, the Sun and Moon.'

At this demand the gods looked grave; for Freia was their dearest treasure. She was the most beautiful maid who ever lived, the light and life of heaven, and if she should leave Asgard, joy would go with her; while the Sun and Moon were the light and life of the Æsir's children, men, who lived in the little world below. But Loki the sly whispered that they would be safe enough if they made another condition on their part, so hard that the builder could not fulfil it. After thinking cautiously, he spoke for them all.

'Mighty man,' quoth he, 'we are willing to agree to your price – upon one condition. It is too long a time that you ask; we cannot wait three half-years for our castle; that is equal to three centuries when one is in a hurry. See that you finish the fort without help in one winter, one short winter, and you shall have fair Freia with the Sun and Moon. But if, on the first day of summer, one stone is wanting to the walls, or if any one has given you aid in the building, then your reward is lost, and you shall depart without payment.' So spoke Loki, in the name of all the gods; but the plan was his own.

At first the stranger shook his head and frowned, saying that in so short a time no one unaided could complete the undertaking. At last he made another offer. 'Let me have but my good horse to help me, and I will try,' he urged. 'Let me bring the useful Svadilföri with me to the task, and I will finish the work in one winter of short days, or lose my reward. Surely, you will not deny me this little help, from one four-footed friend.'

Then again the Æsir consulted, and the wiser of them were doubtful whether it were best to accept the stranger's offer so strangely made. But again Loki urged them to accept. 'Surely, there is no harm,' he said. 'Even with his old horse to help him, he cannot build the castle in the promised time. We shall gain a fortress without trouble and with never a price to pay.'

Loki was so eager that, although the other Æsir did not like this crafty way of making bargains, they finally consented. Then in the presence of the heroes, with the Valkyries and Mimer's head for witnesses, the stranger and the Æsir gave solemn promise that the bargain should be kept.

On the first day of winter the strange builder began his work, and wondrous was the way he set about it. His strength seemed as the strength of a hundred men. As for his horse Svadilföri, he did more work by half than even the mighty builder. In the night he dragged the enormous rocks that were to be used in building the castle, rocks as big as mountains of the earth; while in the daytime the stranger piled them into place with his iron arms. The Æsir watched him with amazement; never was seen such strength in Asgard. Neither Týr the stout nor Thor the strong could match the power of the stranger. The gods began to look at one another uneasily. Who was this mighty one who had come among them, and what if after all he should win his reward? Freia trembled in her palace, and the Sun and Moon grew dim with fear.

Still the work went on, and the fort was piling higher and higher, by day and by night. There were but three days left before the end of winter, and already the building was so tall and so strong that it was safe from the attacks of any giant. The Æsir were delighted with their fine new castle; but their pride was dimmed by the fear that it must be paid for at all too costly a price. For only the gateway remained to be completed, and unless the stranger should fail to finish that in the next three days, they must give him Freia with the Sun and Moon.

The Æsir held a meeting upon Ida Plain, a meeting full of fear and anger. At last they realized what they had done; they had made a bargain with one of the giants, their enemies; and if he won the prize, it would mean sorrow and darkness in heaven and upon earth. 'How did we happen to agree to so mad a bargain?' they asked one another. 'Who suggested the wicked plan which bids fair to cost us all that we most cherish?' Then they remembered that it was Loki who had made the plan; it was he who had insisted that it be carried out and they blamed him for all the trouble.

'It is your counsels, Loki, that have brought this danger upon us,' quoth Father Odin, frowning. 'You chose the way of guile, which is not our way. It now remains for you to help us by guile, if you can. But if you cannot save for us Freia and the Sun and Moon, you shall die. This is my word.' All the other Æsir agreed that this was just. Thor alone was away hunting evil demons at the other end of the world, so he did not know what was going on, and what dangers were threatening Asgard.

Loki was much frightened at the word of All-Father. 'It was my fault,' he cried, 'but how was I to know that he was a giant? He had disguised himself so that he seemed but a strong man. And as for his horse – it looks much like that of other folk. If it were not for the horse, he could not finish the work. Ha! I have a thought! The builder shall not finish the gate; the giant shall not receive his payment. I will cheat the fellow.'

Now it was the last night of winter, and there remained but a few stones to put in place on the top of the wondrous gateway. The giant was sure of his prize, and chuckled to himself as he went out with his horse to drag the remaining stones; for he did not know that the Æsir had guessed at last who he was, and that Loki was plotting to outwit him. Hardly had he gone to work when out of the wood came running a pretty little mare, who neighed to Svadilföri as if inviting the tired horse to leave his work and come to the green fields for a holiday.

Svadilföri, you must remember, had been working hard all winter, with never a sight of four-footed creature of his kind, and he was very lonesome and tired of dragging stones. Giving a snort of disobedience, off he ran after this new friend towards the grassy meadows. Off went the giant after him, howling with rage, and running for dear life, as he saw not only his horse but his chance of success slipping out of reach. It was a mad chase, and all Asgard thundered with the noise of galloping hoofs and the giant's mighty tread. The mare who raced ahead was Loki in disguise, and he led Svadilföri far out of reach, to a hidden meadow that he knew; so that the giant howled and panted up and down all night long, without catching even a sight of his horse.

Now when the morning came the gateway was still unfinished, and night and winter had ended at the same hour. The giant's time was over, and he had forfeited his reward. The Æsir came flocking to the gateway, and how they laughed and triumphed when they found three stones wanting to complete the gate!

'You have failed, fellow,' judged Father Odin sternly, 'and no price shall we pay for work that is still undone. You have failed. Leave Asgard quickly; we have seen all we want of you and of your race.'

Then the giant knew that he was discovered, and he was mad with rage. 'It was a trick!' he bellowed, assuming his own proper form, which was huge as a mountain, and towered high beside the fortress that he had built. 'It was a wicked trick. You shall pay for this in one way or another. I cannot tear down the castle which, ungrateful ones, I have built you, stronger than the strength of any giant. But I will demolish the rest of your shining city!' Indeed, he would have done so in his mighty rage; but at this moment Thor, whom Heimdal had called from the end of the earth by one blast of the golden horn, came rushing to the rescue, drawn in his chariot of goats. Thor jumped to the ground close beside the giant, and before that huge fellow knew what had happened, his head was rolling upon the ground at Father Odin's feet; for with one blow Thor had put an end to the giant's wickedness and had saved Asgard.

'This is the reward you deserve!' Thor cried. 'Not Freia nor the Sun and Moon, but the death that I have in store for all the enemies of the Æsir.'

In this extraordinary way the noble city of Asgard was made safe and complete by the addition of a fortress which no one, not even the giant who built it, could injure, it was so wonder-strong. But always at the top of the gate were lacking three great stones that no one was mighty enough to lift. This was a reminder to the Æsir that now they had the race of giants for their everlasting enemies. And though Loki's trick had saved them Freia, and for the world the Sun and Moon, it was the beginning of trouble in Asgard which lasted as long as Loki lived to make mischief with his guile.

A MIDSUMMER NIGHT'S DREAM

Edith Nesbit

Hermia and Lysander were lovers; but Hermia's father wished her to marry another man, named Demetrius.

Now, in Athens, where they lived, there was a wicked law, by which any girl who refused to marry according to her father's wishes, might be put to death. Hermia's father was so angry with her for refusing to do as he wished, that he actually brought her before the Duke of Athens to ask that she might be killed, if she still refused to obey him. The Duke gave her four days to think about it, and, at the end of that time, if she still refused to marry Demetrius, she would have to die.

Lysander of course was nearly mad with grief, and the best thing to do seemed to him for Hermia to run away to his aunt's house at a place beyond the reach of that cruel law; and there he would come to her and marry her. But before she started, she told her friend, Helena, what she was going to do.

Helena had been Demetrius' sweetheart long before his marriage with Hermia had been thought of, and being very silly, like all jealous people, she could not see that it was not poor Hermia's fault that Demetrius wished to marry her instead of his own lady, Helena. She knew that if she told Demetrius that Hermia was going, as she was, to the wood outside Athens, he would follow her, 'and I can follow him, and at least I shall see him,' she said to herself. So she went to him, and betrayed her friend's secret.

Now this wood where Lysander was to meet Hermia, and where the other two had decided to follow them, was full of fairies, as most woods are, if one only had the eyes to see them, and in this wood on this night were the King and Queen of the fairies, Oberon and Titania. Now fairies are very wise people, but now and then they can be quite as foolish as mortal folk. Oberon and Titania, who might have been as happy as the days were long, had thrown away all their joy in a foolish quarrel. They never met without saying disagreeable things to each other, and scolded each other so dreadfully that all their little fairy followers, for fear, would creep into acorn cups and hide them there.

So, instead of keeping one happy Court and dancing all night through in the moonlight as is fairies' use, the King with his attendants wandered through one part of the wood, while the Queen with hers kept state in another. And the cause of all this trouble was a little boy whom Titania had taken to be one of her followers. Oberon wanted the child to follow him and be one of his fairy knights; but the Queen would not give him up.

On this night, in a mossy moonlit glade, the King and Queen of the fairies met.

'Ill met by moonlight, proud Titania,' said the King.

'What! jealous, Oberon?' answered the Queen. 'You spoil everything with your quarrelling. Come, fairies, let us leave him. I am not friends with him now.'

'It rests with you to make up the quarrel,' said the King.

'Give me that boy, and I will again be your humble servant and suitor.'

'Set your mind at rest,' said the Queen. 'Your whole fairy kingdom buys not that boy from me. Come, fairies.'

And she and her train rode off down the moonbeams.

'Well, go your ways,' said Oberon. 'But I'll be even with you before you leave this wood.'

Then Oberon called his favourite fairy, Puck. Puck was the spirit of mischief. He used to slip into the dairies and take the cream away, and get into the churn so that the butter would not come, and turn the beer sour, and lead people out of their way on dark nights and then laugh at them, and tumble people's stools from under them when they were going to sit down, and upset their hot ale over their chins when they were going to drink.

'Now,' said Oberon to this little sprite, 'fetch me the flower called Love-in-idleness. The juice of that little purple flower laid on the eyes of those who sleep will make them, when they wake, to love the first thing they see. I will put some of the juice of that flower on my Titania's eyes, and when she wakes she will love the first thing she sees, were it lion, bear or wolf, or bull, or meddling monkey, or a busy ape.'

While Puck was gone, Demetrius passed through the glade followed by poor Helena, and still she told him how she loved him and reminded him of all his promises, and still he told her that he did not and could not love her, and that his promises were nothing. Oberon was sorry for poor Helena, and when Puck returned with the flower, he bade him follow Demetrius and put some of the juice on his eyes, so that he might love Helena when he woke and looked on her, as much as she loved him. So Puck set off, and wandering through the wood found, not Demetrius, but Lysander, on whose eyes he put the juice; but when Lysander woke, he saw not his own Hermia, but Helena, who was walking through the wood looking for the cruel Demetrius; and directly he saw her he loved her and left his own lady, under the spell of the purple flower.

When Hermia woke she found Lysander gone, and wandered

about the wood trying to find him. Puck went back and told Oberon what he had done, and Oberon soon found that he had made a mistake, and set about looking for Demetrius, and having found him, put some of the juice on his eyes. And the first thing Demetrius saw when he woke was also Helena. So now Demetrius and Lysander were both following her through the wood, and it was Hermia's turn to follow her lover as Helena had done before. The end of it was that Helena and Hermia began to quarrel, and Demetrius and Lysander went off to fight. Oberon was very sorry to see his kind scheme to help these lovers turn out so badly. So he said to Puck—

'These two young men are going to fight. You must overhang the night with drooping fog, and lead them so astray, that one will never find the other. When they are tired out, they will fall asleep. Then drop this other herb on Lysander's eyes. That will give him his old sight and his old love. Then each man will have the lady who loves him, and they will all think that this has been only a Midsummer Night's Dream. Then when this is done, all will be well with them.'

So Puck went and did as he was told, and when the two had fallen asleep without meeting each other, Puck poured the juice on Lysander's eyes, and said:—

> 'When thou wakest,
> Thou takest
> True delight
> In the sight
> Of thy former lady's eye:
> Jack shall have Jill;
> Nought shall go ill.'

Meanwhile Oberon found Titania asleep on a bank where grew wild thyme, oxlips and violets, and woodbine, musk-roses and eglantine. There Titania always slept a part of the night, wrapped in the enamelled skin of a snake. Oberon stooped over her and laid the juice on her eyes, saying:—

'What thou seest when thou wake,
Do it for thy true love take.'

Now, it happened that when Titania woke the first thing she saw was a stupid clown, one of a party of players who had come out into the wood to rehearse their play. This clown had met with Puck, who had clapped an ass's head on his shoulders so that it looked as if it grew there. Directly Titania woke and saw this dreadful monster, she said, 'What angel is this? Are you as wise as you are beautiful?'

'If I am wise enough to find my way out of this wood, that's enough for me,' said the foolish clown.

'Do not desire to go out of the wood,' said Titania. The spell of the love-juice was on her, and to her the clown seemed the most beautiful and delightful creature on all the earth. 'I love you,' she went on. 'Come with me, and I will give you fairies to attend on you.'

So she called four fairies, whose names were Peaseblossom, Cobweb, Moth and Mustardseed.

'You must attend this gentleman,' said the Queen. 'Feed him with apricots and dewberries, purple grapes, green figs and mulberries. Steal honey-bags for him from the bumble-bees, and with the wings of painted butterflies fan the moonbeams from his sleeping eyes.'

'I will,' said one of the fairies, and all the others said, 'I will.'

'Now, sit down with me,' said the Queen to the clown, 'and let me stroke your dear cheeks, and stick musk-roses in your smooth, sleek head, and kiss your fair large ears, my gentle joy.'

'Where's Peaseblossom?' asked the clown with the ass's head.

He did not care much about the Queen's affection, but he was very proud of having fairies to wait on him. 'Ready,' said Peaseblossom.

'Scratch my head, Peaseblossom,' said the clown. 'Where's Cobweb?' 'Ready,' said Cobweb.

'Kill me,' said the clown, 'the red bumble-bee on the top of the thistle yonder, and bring me the honey-bag. Where's Mustardseed?'

'Ready,' said Mustardseed.

'Oh, I want nothing,' said the clown. 'Only just help Cobweb to scratch. I must go to the barber's, for methinks I am marvellous hairy about the face.'

'Would you like anything to eat?' said the fairy Queen.

'I should like some good dry oats,' said the clown – for his donkey's head made him desire donkey's food – 'and some hay to follow.'

'Shall some of my fairies fetch you new nuts from the squirrel's house?' asked the Queen.

'I'd rather have a handful or two of good dried peas,' said the clown. 'But please don't let any of your people disturb me; I am going to sleep.'

Then said the Queen, 'And I will wind thee in my arms.'

And so when Oberon came along he found his beautiful Queen lavishing kisses and endearments on a clown with a donkey's head.

And before he released her from the enchantment, he persuaded her to give him the child he so much desired to have. Then he took pity on her, and threw some juice of the disenchanting flower on her pretty eyes; and then in a moment she saw plainly the donkey-headed clown she had been loving, and knew how foolish she had been.

Oberon took off the ass's head from the clown, and left him to finish his sleep with his own silly head lying on the thyme and violets.

Thus all was made plain and straight again. Oberon and Titania loved each other more than ever. Demetrius thought of no one but Helena, and Helena had never had any thought of anyone but Demetrius.

As for Hermia and Lysander, they were as loving a couple as you could meet in a day's march, even through a fairy wood.

So the four mortal lovers went back to Athens and were married; and the fairy King and Queen live happily together in that very wood at this very day.

SOLITUDE – AN EXCERPT FROM *WALDEN*

Henry David Thoreau

This is a delicious evening, when the whole body is one sense, and imbibes delight through every pore. I go and come with a strange liberty in Nature, a part of herself. As I walk along the stony shore of the pond in my shirt sleeves, though it is cool as well as cloudy and windy, and I see nothing special to attract me, all the elements are unusually congenial to me. The bullfrogs trump to usher in the night, and the note of the whippoorwill is borne on the rippling wind from over the water. Sympathy with the fluttering alder and poplar leaves almost takes away my breath; yet, like the lake, my serenity is rippled but not ruffled. These small waves raised by the evening wind are as remote from storm as the smooth reflecting surface. Though it is now dark, the wind still blows and roars in the wood, the waves still dash and some creatures lull the rest with their notes. The repose is never complete. The wildest animals do not repose, but seek their prey now; the fox, and skunk, and rabbit, now roam the fields and woods without fear. They are Nature's watchmen – links which connect the days of animated life.

When I return to my house I find that visitors have been there and left their cards, either a bunch of flowers, or a wreath of evergreen, or a name in pencil on a yellow walnut leaf or a chip. They who come rarely to the woods take some little piece of the forest into their hands to play with by the way, which they leave, either intentionally or accidentally. One has peeled a willow wand, woven it into a ring and dropped it on my table. I could always tell if visitors had called in my absence, either by the bended twigs or grass, or the print of their shoes, and generally of what sex or age or quality they were by some slight trace left, as a flower dropped, or a bunch of grass plucked and thrown away, even as far off as the railroad, half a mile distant, or by the lingering odour of a cigar or pipe. Nay, I was frequently notified of the passage of a traveller along the highway sixty rods off by the scent of his pipe.

There is commonly sufficient space about us. Our horizon is never quite at our elbows. The thick wood is not just at our door, nor the pond, but somewhat is always clearing, familiar and worn by us, appropriated and fenced in some way, and reclaimed from Nature. For what reason have I this vast range and circuit, some square miles of unfrequented forest, for my privacy, abandoned to me by men? My nearest neighbour is a mile distant, and no house is visible from any place but the hill-tops within half a mile of my own. I have my horizon bounded by woods all to myself; a distant view of the railroad where it touches the pond on the one hand, and of the fence which skirts the woodland road on the other. But for the most part it is as solitary where I live as on the prairies. It is as much Asia or Africa as New England. I have, as it were, my own sun and moon and stars, and a little world all to myself. At night there was never a traveller passed my house, or knocked at my door, more than if I were the first or last man; unless it were in the spring, when at long intervals some came from the village to fish for pouts – they plainly fished much more in the Walden Pond of their own natures, and baited their hooks with darkness – but they soon retreated, usually with light baskets, and left 'the world to darkness and to me', and the black kernel of the night was never profaned by any human neighbourhood. I believe that men are generally still a little afraid of the dark, though Christianity and candles have been introduced.

Yet I experienced sometimes that the most sweet and tender, the most innocent and encouraging society may be found in any natural object, even for the poor misanthrope and most melancholy man. There can be no very black melancholy to him who lives in the midst of Nature and has his senses still. There was never yet such a storm but it was Æolian music to a healthy and innocent ear. Nothing can rightly compel a simple and brave man to a vulgar sadness. While I enjoy the friendship of the seasons I trust that nothing can make life a burden to me. The gentle rain which waters my beans and keeps me in the house to-day is not drear and melancholy, but good for me too. Though it prevents my hoeing them, it is of far more worth than my hoeing. If it should continue so long as to cause the seeds to rot in the ground and destroy the potatoes in the low lands, it would still be good for the grass on the uplands, and, being good for the grass, it would be good for me. Sometimes, when I compare myself with other men, it seems as if I were more favoured by the gods than they, beyond any deserts that I am conscious of; as if I had a warrant and surety at their hands which my fellows have not, and were especially guided and guarded. I do not flatter myself, but if it be possible they flatter me. I have never felt lonesome, or in the least oppressed by a sense of solitude, but once, and that was a few weeks after I came to the woods, when, for an hour, I doubted if the near neighbourhood of man was not essential to a serene and healthy life. To be alone was something unpleasant. But I was at the same time conscious of a slight insanity in my mood, and seemed to foresee my recovery. In the midst of a gentle rain while these thoughts prevailed, I was suddenly sensible of such sweet and beneficent society in Nature, in the very pattering of the drops, and in every sound and sight around my house, an infinite and unaccountable friendliness all at once like an atmosphere sustaining me, as made the fancied advantages of human neighbourhood insignificant, and I have never thought of them since. Every little pine needle expanded and swelled with sympathy and befriended me. I was so distinctly made aware of the presence of something kindred to me, even in scenes which we are accustomed to call wild and dreary, and also that the nearest of blood to me and humanest was not a person nor a villager, that I thought no place could ever be strange to me again.—

> 'Mourning untimely consumes the sad;
> Few are their days in the land of the living,
> Beautiful daughter of Toscar.'

Some of my pleasantest hours were during the long rain storms in the spring or fall, which confined me to the house for the afternoon as well as the forenoon, soothed by their ceaseless roar and pelting; when an early twilight ushered in a long evening in which many thoughts had time to take root and unfold themselves. In those driving north-east rains which tried the village houses so, when the maids stood ready with mop and pail in front entries to keep the deluge out, I sat behind my door in my little house, which was all entry, and thoroughly enjoyed its protection. In one heavy thunder shower the lightning struck a large pitch-pine across the pond, making a very conspicuous and perfectly regular spiral groove from top to bottom, an inch or more deep, and four or five inches wide, as you would groove a walking-stick. I passed it again the other day, and was struck with awe on looking up and beholding that mark, now more distinct than ever, where a terrific and resistless bolt came down out of the harmless sky eight years ago. Men frequently say to me, 'I should think you would feel lonesome down there, and want to be nearer to folks, rainy and snowy days and nights especially.' I am tempted to reply to such – This whole earth which we inhabit is but a point in space. How far apart, think you, dwell the two most distant inhabitants of yonder star, the breadth of whose disc cannot be appreciated by our instruments? Why should I feel lonely? is not our planet in the Milky Way? This which you put seems to me not to be the most important question. What sort of space is that which separates a man from his fellows and makes him solitary? I have found that no exertion of the legs can bring two minds much nearer to one another. What do we want most to dwell near to? Not to many men surely, the depot, the post-office, the bar-room, the meeting-house, the school-house, the grocery, Beacon Hill or the Five Points, where men most congregate, but to the perennial source of our life, whence in all our experience we have found that to issue, as the willow stands near the water and sends out its roots in that direction. This will vary with different natures, but this is the place where a wise man will dig his cellar . . . I one evening overtook one of my townsmen, who has accumulated what is called 'a handsome property' – though I never got a *fair* view of it – on the Walden road, driving a pair of cattle to market, who inquired of me how I could bring my mind to give up so many of the comforts of life. I answered that I was very sure I liked it passably well; I was not joking. And so I went home to my bed, and left him to pick his way through the darkness and the mud to Brighton – or Bright-town – which place he would reach some time in the morning.

Any prospect of awakening or coming to life to a dead man makes indifferent all times and places. The place where that may occur is always the same, and indescribably pleasant to all our senses. For the most part we allow only outlying and transient circumstances to make our occasions. They are, in fact, the cause of our distraction.

Nearest to all things is that power which fashions their being. *Next* to us the grandest laws are continually being executed. *Next* to us is not the workman whom we have hired, with whom we love so well to talk, but the workman whose work we are.

'How vast and profound is the influence of the subtile powers of Heaven and of Earth!'

'We seek to perceive them, and we do not see them; we seek to hear them, and we do not hear them; identified with the substance of things, they cannot be separated from them.'

'They cause that in all the universe men purify and sanctify their hearts, and clothe themselves in their holiday garments to offer sacrifices and oblations to their ancestors. It is an ocean of subtile intelligences. They are every where, above us, on our left, on our right; they environ us on all sides.'

We are the subjects of an experiment which is not a little interesting to me. Can we not do without the society of our gossips a little while under these circumstances – have our own thoughts to cheer us? Confucius says truly, 'Virtue does not remain as an abandoned orphan; it must of necessity have neighbours.'

With thinking we may be beside ourselves in a sane sense. By a conscious effort of the mind we can stand aloof from actions and their consequences; and all things, good and bad, go by us like a torrent. We are not wholly involved in Nature. I may be either the drift-wood in the stream, or Indra in the sky looking down on it. I *may* be affected by a theatrical exhibition; on the other hand, I *may not* be affected by an actual event which appears to concern me much more. I only know myself as a human entity; the scene, so to speak, of thoughts and affections; and am sensible of a certain doubleness by which I can stand as remote from myself as from another. However intense my experience, I am conscious of the presence and criticism of a part of me, which, as it were, is not a part of me, but spectator, sharing no experience, but taking note of it; and that is no more I than it is you. When the play, it may be the tragedy, of life is over, the spectator goes his way. It was a kind of fiction, a work of the imagination only, so far as he was concerned. This doubleness may easily make us poor neighbours and friends sometimes.

I find it wholesome to be alone the greater part of the time. To be in company, even with the best, is soon wearisome and dissipating. I love to be alone. I never found the companion that was so companionable as solitude. We are for the most part more lonely when we go abroad among men than when we stay in our chambers. A man thinking or working is always alone, let him be where he will. Solitude is not measured by the miles of space that intervene between a man and his fellows. The really diligent student in one of the crowded hives of Cambridge College is as solitary as a dervish in the desert. The farmer can work alone in the field or the woods all day, hoeing or chopping, and not feel lonesome, because he is employed; but when he comes home at night he cannot sit down in a room alone, at the mercy of his thoughts, but must be where he can 'see the folks', and recreate, and as he thinks remunerate himself for his day's solitude; and hence he wonders how the student can sit alone in the house all night and most of the day without ennui and 'the blues'; but he does not realize that the student, though in the house, is still at work in *his* field, and chopping in his woods, as the farmer in his, and in turn seeks the same recreation and society that the latter does, though it may be a more condensed form of it.

Society is commonly too cheap. We meet at very short intervals, not having had time to acquire any new value for each other. We meet at meals three times a day, and give each other a new taste of that old musty cheese that we are. We have had to agree on a certain set of rules, called etiquette and politeness, to make this frequent meeting tolerable and that we need not come to open war. We meet at the post-office, and at the sociable, and about the fireside every night; we live thick and are in each other's way, and stumble over one another, and I think that we thus lose some respect for one another. Certainly less frequency would suffice for all important and hearty communications. Consider the girls in a factory – never alone, hardly in their dreams. It would be better if there were but one inhabitant to a square mile, as where I live. The value of a man is not in his skin, that we should touch him.

I have heard of a man lost in the woods and dying of famine and exhaustion at the foot of a tree, whose loneliness was relieved by the grotesque visions with which, owing to bodily weakness, his diseased imagination surrounded him, and which he believed to be real. So also, owing to bodily and mental health and strength, we may be continually cheered by a like but more normal and natural society, and come to know that we are never alone.

I have a great deal of company in my house; especially in the morning, when nobody calls. Let me suggest a few comparisons, that some one may convey an idea of my situation. I am no more lonely than the loon in the pond that laughs so loud, or than Walden Pond itself. What company has that lonely lake, I pray? And yet it has not the blue devils, but the blue angels in it, in the azure tint of its waters. The sun is alone, except in thick weather, when there sometimes appear to be two, but one is a mock sun. God is alone – but the devil, he is far from being alone; he sees a great deal of company; he is legion. I am no more lonely than a single mullein or dandelion in a pasture, or a bean leaf, or sorrel, or a horse-fly, or a bumble-bee. I am no more lonely than the Mill Brook, or a weathercock, or the north star, or the south wind, or an April shower, or a January thaw, or the first spider in a new house.

I have occasional visits in the long winter evenings, when the snow falls fast and the wind howls in the wood, from an old settler and original proprietor, who is reported to have dug Walden Pond, and stoned it, and fringed it with pine woods; who tells me stories of old time and of new eternity; and between us we manage to pass a cheerful evening with social mirth and pleasant views of things, even without apples or cider – a most wise and humorous friend, whom I love much, who keeps himself more secret than ever did Goffe or Whalley; and though he is thought to be dead, none can show where he is buried. An elderly dame, too, dwells in my neighbourhood, invisible to most persons, in whose odorous herb garden I love to stroll sometimes, gathering simples and listening to her fables; for she has a genius of unequalled fertility, and her memory runs back farther than mythology, and she can tell me the original of every fable, and on what fact every one is founded, for the incidents occurred when she was young. A ruddy and lusty old dame, who delights in all weathers and seasons, and is likely to outlive all her children yet.

The indescribable innocence and beneficence of Nature – of sun and wind and rain, of summer and winter – such health, such cheer, they afford forever! and such sympathy have they ever with our race, that all Nature would be affected, and the sun's brightness fade, and the winds would sigh humanely, and the clouds rain tears, and the woods shed their leaves and put on mourning in midsummer, if any man should ever for a just cause grieve. Shall I not have intelligence with the earth? Am I not partly leaves and vegetable mould myself?

What is the pill which will keep us well, serene, contented? Not my or thy great-grandfather's, but our great-grandmother Nature's universal, vegetable, botanic medicines, by which she has kept herself young always, outlived so many old Parrs in her day, and fed her health with their decaying fatness. For my panacea, instead of one of those quack vials of a mixture dipped from Acheron and the Dead Sea, which come out of those long shallow black-schooner looking wagons which we sometimes see made to carry bottles, let me have a draught of undiluted morning air. Morning air! If men will not drink of this at the fountain-head of the day, why, then, we must even bottle up some and sell it in the shops, for the benefit of those who have lost their subscription ticket to morning time in this world. But remember, it will not keep quite till noon-day even in the coolest cellar, but drive out the stopples long ere that and follow westward the steps of Aurora. I am no worshipper of Hygeia, who was the daughter of that old herb-doctor Æsculapius, and who is represented on monuments holding a serpent in one hand, and in the other a cup out of which the serpent sometimes drinks; but rather of Hebe, cupbearer to Jupiter, who was the daughter of Juno and wild lettuce, and who had the power of restoring gods and men to the vigour of youth. She was probably the only thoroughly sound-conditioned, healthy and robust young lady that ever walked the globe, and wherever she came it was spring.

A SOCIETY

Virginia Woolf

This is how it all came about. Six or seven of us were sitting one day after tea. Some were gazing across the street into the windows of a milliner's shop where the light still shone brightly upon scarlet feathers and golden slippers. Others were idly occupied in building little towers of sugar upon the edge of the tea tray. After a time, so far as I can remember, we drew round the fire and began as usual to praise men – how strong, how noble, how brilliant, how courageous, how beautiful they were – how we envied those who by hook or by crook managed to get attached to one for life – when Poll, who had said nothing, burst into tears. Poll, I must tell you, has always been queer. For one thing her father was a strange man. He left her a fortune in his will, but on condition that she read all the books in the London Library. We comforted her as best we could; but we knew in our hearts how vain it was. For though we like her, Poll is no beauty; leaves her shoe laces untied; and must have been thinking, while we praised men, that not one of them would ever wish to marry her. At last she dried her tears. For some time we could make nothing of what she said. Strange enough it was in all conscience. She told us that, as we knew, she spent most of her time in the London Library, reading. She had begun, she said, with English literature on the top floor; and was steadily working her way down to *The Times* on the bottom. And now half, or perhaps only a quarter, way through a terrible thing had happened. She could read no more. Books were not what we thought them. 'Books,' she cried, rising to her feet and speaking with an intensity of desolation which I shall never forget, 'are for the most part unutterably bad!'

Of course we cried out that Shakespeare wrote books, and Milton and Shelley.

'Oh, yes,' she interrupted us. 'You've been well taught, I can see. But you are not members of the London Library.' Here her sobs broke forth anew. At length, recovering a little, she opened one of the pile of books which she always carried about with her – 'From a Window' or 'In a Garden', or some such name as that it was called, and it was written by a man called Benton or Henson, or something of that kind. She read the first few pages. We listened in silence. 'But that's not a book,' someone said. So she chose another. This time it was a history, but I have forgotten the writer's name. Our trepidation increased as she went on. Not a word of it seemed to be true, and the style in which it was written was execrable.

'Poetry! Poetry!' we cried, impatiently. 'Read us poetry!' I cannot describe the desolation which fell upon us as she opened a little volume and mouthed out the verbose, sentimental foolery which it contained.

'It must have been written by a woman,' one of us urged. But no. She told us that it was written by a young man, one of the most famous poets of the day. I leave you to imagine what the shock of the discovery was. Though we all cried and begged her to read no more, she persisted and read us extracts from the Lives of the Lord Chancellors. When she had finished, Jane, the eldest and wisest of us, rose to her feet and said that she for one was not convinced.

'Why,' she asked, 'if men write such rubbish as this, should our mothers have wasted their youth in bringing them into the world?'

We were all silent; and, in the silence, poor Poll could be heard sobbing out, 'Why, why did my father teach me to read?'

Clorinda was the first to come to her senses. 'It's all our fault,' she said. 'Every one of us knows how to read. But no one, save Poll, has ever taken the trouble to do it. I, for one, have taken it for granted that it was a woman's duty to spend her youth in bearing children. I venerated my mother for bearing ten; still more my grandmother for bearing fifteen; it was, I confess, my own ambition to bear twenty. We have gone on all these ages supposing that men were equally industrious, and that their works were of equal merit. While we have borne the children, they, we supposed, have borne the books and the pictures. We have populated the world. They have civilized it. But now that we can read, what prevents us from judging the results? Before we bring another child into the world we must swear that we will find out what the world is like.'

So we made ourselves into a society for asking questions. One of us was to visit a man-of-war; another was to hide herself in a scholar's study; another was to attend a meeting of business men; while all were to read books, look at pictures, go to concerts, keep our eyes open in the streets and ask questions perpetually. We were very young. You can judge of our simplicity when I tell you that before parting that night we agreed that the objects of life were to produce good people and good books. Our questions were to be directed to finding out how far these objects were now attained by men. We vowed solemnly that we would not bear a single child until we were satisfied.

Off we went then, some to the British Museum; others to the King's Navy; some to Oxford; others to Cambridge; we visited the Royal Academy and the Tate; heard modern music in concert rooms, went to the Law Courts and saw new plays. No one dined out without asking her partner certain questions and carefully noting his replies. At intervals we met together and compared our observations. Oh, those were merry meetings! Never have I laughed so much as I did when Rose read her notes upon 'Honour' and described how she had dressed herself as an Æthiopian Prince and gone aboard one of His Majesty's ships. Discovering the hoax, the Captain visited her (now disguised as a private gentleman) and demanded that honour should be satisfied. 'But how?' she asked. 'How?' he bellowed. 'With the cane of course!' Seeing that he was beside himself with rage and expecting that her last moment had come, she bent over and received, to her amazement, six light taps upon the behind. 'The honour of the British Navy is avenged!' he cried, and, raising herself, she saw him with the sweat pouring down his face holding out a trembling right hand. 'Away!' she exclaimed, striking an attitude and imitating the ferocity of his own expression. 'My honour has still to be satisfied!' 'Spoken like a gentleman!' he returned, and fell into profound thought. 'If six strokes avenge the honour of the King's Navy,' he mused, 'how many avenge the honour of a private gentleman?' He said he would prefer to lay the case before his brother officers. She replied haughtily that she could not wait. He praised her sensibility. 'Let me see,' he cried suddenly, 'did your father keep a carriage?' 'No,' she said. 'Or a riding horse?' 'We had a donkey,' she bethought her, 'which drew the mowing machine.' At this his face lighted. 'My mother's name—' she added. 'For God's sake, man, don't mention your mother's name!' he shrieked, trembling like an aspen and flushing to the roots of his hair, and it was ten minutes at least before she could induce him to proceed. At length he decreed that if she gave him four strokes and a half in the small of the back at a spot indicated by himself (the half conceded, he said, in recognition of the fact that her great grandmother's uncle was killed at Trafalgar) it was his opinion that her honour would be as good as new. This was done; they retired to a restaurant; drank two bottles of wine for which he insisted upon paying; and parted with protestations of eternal friendship.

Then we had Fanny's account of her visit to the Law Courts. At her first visit she had come to the conclusion that the Judges were either made of wood or were impersonated by large animals resembling man who had been trained to move with extreme dignity, mumble and nod their heads. To test her theory she had liberated a handkerchief of bluebottles at the critical moment of a trial, but was unable to judge whether the creatures gave signs of humanity for the buzzing of the flies induced so sound a sleep that she only woke in time to see the prisoners led into the cells below. But from the evidence she brought we voted that it is unfair to suppose that the Judges are men.

Helen went to the Royal Academy, but when asked to deliver her report upon the pictures she began to recite from a pale blue volume, 'O! for the touch of a vanished hand and the sound of a voice that is still. Home is the hunter, home from the hill. He gave his bridle reins a shake. Love is sweet, love is brief. Spring, the fair spring, is the year's pleasant King. O! to be in England now that April's there. Men must work and women must weep. The path of duty is the way to glory—' We could listen to no more of this gibberish.

'We want no more poetry!' we cried.

'Daughters of England!' she began, but here we pulled her down, a vase of water getting spilt over her in the scuffle.

'Thank God!' she exclaimed, shaking herself like a dog. 'Now I'll roll on the carpet and see if I can't brush off what remains of the Union Jack. Then perhaps—' here she rolled energetically. Getting up she began to explain to us what modern pictures are like when Castalia stopped her.

'What is the average size of a picture?' she asked. 'Perhaps two feet by two and a half,' she said. Castalia made notes while Helen spoke, and when she had done, and we were trying not to meet each other's eyes, rose and said, 'At your wish I spent last week at Oxbridge, disguised as a charwoman. I thus had access to the rooms of several Professors and will now attempt to give you some idea – only,' she broke off, 'I can't think how to do it. It's all so queer. These Professors,' she went on, 'live in large houses built round grass plots each in a kind of cell by himself. Yet they have every convenience and comfort. You have only to press a button or light a little lamp. Their papers are beautifully filed. Books abound. There are no children or animals, save half a dozen stray cats and one aged bullfinch – a cock. I remember,' she broke off, 'an Aunt of mine who lived at Dulwich and kept cactuses. You reached the conservatory through the double drawing-room, and there, on the hot pipes, were dozens of them, ugly, squat, bristly little plants each in a separate pot. Once in a hundred years the Aloe flowered, so my Aunt said. But she died before that happened—' We told her to keep to the point. 'Well,' she resumed, 'when Professor Hobkin was out, I examined his life work, an edition of Sappho. It's a queer looking book, six or seven inches thick, not all by Sappho. Oh, no. Most of it is a defence of Sappho's chastity, which some German had denied, and I can assure you the passion with which these two gentlemen argued, the learning they displayed, the prodigious ingenuity with which they disputed the use of some implement which looked to me for all the world like a hairpin astounded me; especially when the door opened and Professor Hobkin himself appeared. A very nice, mild, old gentleman, but what could *he* know about chastity?' We misunderstood her.

'No, no,' she protested, 'he's the soul of honour I'm sure – not that he resembles Rose's sea captain in the least. I was thinking rather of my Aunt's cactuses. What could *they* know about chastity?'

Again we told her not to wander from the point – did the Oxbridge professors help to produce good people and good books? – the objects of life.

'There!' she exclaimed. 'It never struck me to ask. It never occurred to me that they could possibly produce anything.'

'I believe,' said Sue, 'that you made some mistake. Probably Professor Hobkin was a gynæcologist. A scholar is a very different sort of man. A scholar is overflowing with humour and invention – perhaps addicted to wine, but what of that? – a delightful companion, generous, subtle, imaginative – as stands to reason. For he spends his life in company with the finest human beings that have ever existed.'

'Hum,' said Castalia. 'Perhaps I'd better go back and try again.'

Some three months later it happened that I was sitting alone when Castalia entered. I don't know what it was in the look of her that so moved me; but I could not restrain myself, and, dashing across the room, I clasped her in my arms. Not only was she very beautiful; she seemed also in the highest spirits. 'How happy you look!' I exclaimed, as she sat down.

'I've been at Oxbridge,' she said.

'Asking questions?'

'Answering them,' she replied.

'You have not broken our vow?' I said anxiously, noticing something about her figure.

'Oh, the vow,' she said casually. 'I'm going to have a baby, if that's what you mean. You can't imagine,' she burst out, 'how exciting, how beautiful, how satisfying—'

'What is?' I asked.

'To – to – answer questions,' she replied in some confusion. Whereupon she told me the whole of her story. But in the middle of an account which interested and excited me more than anything I had ever heard, she gave the strangest cry, half whoop, half holloa—

'Chastity! Chastity! Where's my chastity!' she cried. 'Help Ho! The scent bottle!'

There was nothing in the room but a cruet containing mustard, which I was about to administer when she recovered her composure.

'You should have thought of that three months ago,' I said severely.

'True,' she replied. 'There's not much good in thinking of it now. It was unfortunate, by the way, that my mother had me called Castalia.'

'Oh, Castalia, your mother—' I was beginning when she reached for the mustard pot.

'No, no, no,' she said, shaking her head. 'If you'd been a chaste woman yourself you would have screamed at the sight of me – instead of which you rushed across the room and took me in your arms. No, Cassandra. We are neither of us chaste.' So we went on talking.

Meanwhile the room was filling up, for it was the day appointed to discuss the results of our observations. Everyone, I thought, felt as I did about Castalia. They kissed her and said how glad they were to see her again. At length, when we were all assembled, Jane rose and said that it was time to begin. She began by saying that we had now asked questions for over five years, and that though the results were bound to be inconclusive – here Castalia nudged me and whispered that she was not so sure about that. Then she got up, and, interrupting Jane in the middle of a sentence, said:

'Before you say any more, I want to know – am I to stay in the room? Because,' she added, 'I have to confess that I am an impure woman.'

Everyone looked at her in astonishment.

'You are going to have a baby?' asked Jane.

She nodded her head.

It was extraordinary to see the different expressions on their faces. A sort of hum went through the room, in which I could catch the words 'impure', 'baby', 'Castalia' and so on. Jane, who was herself considerably moved, put it to us:

'Shall she go? Is she impure?'

Such a roar filled the room as might have been heard in the street outside.

'No! No! No! Let her stay! Impure? Fiddlesticks!' Yet I fancied that some of the youngest, girls of nineteen or twenty, held back as if overcome with shyness. Then we all came about her and began asking questions, and at last I saw one of the youngest, who had kept in the background, approach shyly and say to her:

'What is chastity then? I mean is it good, or is it bad, or is it nothing at all?' She replied so low that I could not catch what she said.

'You know I was shocked,' said another, 'for at least ten minutes.'

'In my opinion,' said Poll, who was growing crusty from always reading in the London Library, 'chastity is nothing but ignorance – a most discreditable state of mind. We should admit only the unchaste to our society. I vote that Castalia shall be our President.'

This was violently disputed.

'It is as unfair to brand women with chastity as with unchastity,' said Poll. 'Some of us haven't the opportunity either. Moreover, I don't believe Cassy herself maintains that she acted as she did from a pure love of knowledge.'

'He is only twenty-one and divinely beautiful,' said Cassy, with a ravishing gesture.

'I move,' said Helen, 'that no one be allowed to talk of chastity or unchastity save those who are in love.'

'Oh, bother,' said Judith, who had been enquiring into scientific matters, 'I'm not in love and I'm longing to explain my measures for dispensing with prostitutes and fertilizing virgins by Act of Parliament.'

She went on to tell us of an invention of hers to be erected at Tube stations and other public resorts, which, upon payment of a small fee, would safeguard the nation's health, accommodate its sons and relieve its daughters. Then she had contrived a method of preserving in sealed tubes the germs of future Lord Chancellors 'or poets or painters or musicians,' she went on, 'supposing, that is to say, that these breeds are not extinct, and that women still wish to bear children—'

'Of course we wish to bear children!' cried Castalia, impatiently. Jane rapped the table.

'That is the very point we are met to consider,' she said. 'For five years we have been trying to find out whether we are justified in continuing the human race. Castalia has anticipated our decision. But it remains for the rest of us to make up our minds.'

Here one after another of our messengers rose and delivered their reports. The marvels of civilization far exceeded our expectations, and, as we learnt for the first time how man flies in the air, talks across space, penetrates to the heart of an atom and embraces the universe in his speculations, a murmur of admiration burst from our lips.

'We are proud,' we cried, 'that our mothers sacrificed their youth in such a cause as this!' Castalia, who had been listening intently, looked prouder than all the rest. Then Jane reminded us that we had still much to learn, and Castalia begged us to make haste. On we went through a vast tangle of statistics. We learnt that England has a population of so many millions, and that such and such a proportion of them is constantly hungry and in prison; that the average size of a working man's family is such, and that so great a percentage of women die from maladies incident to childbirth. Reports were read of visits to factories, shops, slums and dockyards. Descriptions were given of the Stock Exchange, of a gigantic house of business in the City, and of a Government Office. The British Colonies were now discussed, and some account was given of our rule in India, Africa and Ireland. I was sitting by Castalia and I noticed her uneasiness.

'We shall never come to any conclusion at all at this rate,' she said. 'As it appears that civilization is so much more complex than we had any notion, would it not be better to confine ourselves to our original enquiry? We agreed that it was the object of life to produce good people and good books. All this time we have been talking of aeroplanes, factories and money. Let us talk about men themselves and their arts, for that is the heart of the matter.'

So the diners out stepped forward with long slips of paper containing answers to their questions. These had been framed after much consideration. A good man, we had agreed, must at any rate be honest, passionate and unworldly. But whether or not a particular man possessed those qualities could only be discovered by asking questions, often beginning at a remote distance from the centre. Is Kensington a nice place to live in? Where is your son being educated – and your daughter? Now please tell me, what do you pay for your cigars? By the way, is Sir Joseph a baronet or only a knight? Often it seemed that we learnt more from trivial questions of this kind than from more direct ones. 'I accepted my peerage,' said Lord Bunkum, 'because my wife wished it.' I forget how many titles were accepted for the same reason. 'Working fifteen hours out of the twenty-four, as I do—' ten thousand professional men began.

'No, no, of course you can neither read nor write. But why do you work so hard?' 'My dear lady, with a growing family—' 'But *why* does your family grow?' Their wives wished that too, or perhaps it was the British Empire. But more significant than the answers were the refusals to answer. Very few would reply at all to questions about morality and religion, and such answers as were given were not serious. Questions as to the value of money and power were almost invariably brushed aside, or pressed at extreme risk to the asker. 'I'm sure,' said Jill, 'that if Sir Harley Tightboots hadn't been carving the mutton when I asked him about the capitalist system he would have cut my throat. The only reason why we escaped with our lives over and over again is that men are at once so hungry and so chivalrous. They despise us too much to mind what we say.'

'Of course they despise us,' said Eleanor. 'At the same time how do you account for this – I made enquiries among the artists. Now, no woman has ever been an artist, has she, Poll?'

'Jane–Austen–Charlotte–Brontë–George–Eliot,' cried Poll, like a man crying muffins in a back street.

'Damn the woman!' someone exclaimed. 'What a bore she is!'

'Since Sappho there has been no female of first rate—' Eleanor began, quoting from a weekly newspaper.

'It's now well known that Sappho was the somewhat lewd invention of Professor Hobkin,' Ruth interrupted.

'Anyhow, there is no reason to suppose that any woman ever has been able to write or ever will be able to write,' Eleanor continued. 'And yet, whenever I go among authors they never cease to talk to me about their books. Masterly! I say, or Shakespeare himself! (for one must say something) and I assure you, they believe me.'

'That proves nothing,' said Jane. 'They all do it. Only,' she sighed, 'it doesn't seem to help *us* much. Perhaps we had better examine modern literature next. Liz, it's your turn.'

Elizabeth rose and said that in order to prosecute her enquiry she had dressed as a man and been taken for a reviewer.

'I have read new books pretty steadily for the past five years,' said she. 'Mr Wells is the most popular living writer; then comes Mr Arnold Bennett; then Mr Compton Mackenzie; Mr McKenna and Mr Walpole may be bracketed together.' She sat down.

'But you've told us nothing!' we expostulated. 'Or do you mean that these gentlemen have greatly surpassed Jane–Eliot and that English fiction is – where's that review of yours? Oh, yes, "safe in their hands".'

'Safe, quite safe,' she said, shifting uneasily from foot to foot. 'And I'm sure that they give away even more than they receive.'

We were all sure of that. 'But,' we pressed her, 'do they write good books?'

'Good books?' she said, looking at the ceiling. 'You must remember,' she began, speaking with extreme rapidity, 'that fiction is the mirror of life. And you can't deny that education is of the highest importance, and that it would be extremely annoying, if you found yourself alone at Brighton late at night, not to know which was the best boarding house to stay at, and suppose it was a dripping Sunday evening – wouldn't it be nice to go to the Movies?'

'But what has that got to do with it?' we asked.

'Nothing – nothing – nothing whatever,' she replied.

'Well, tell us the truth,' we bade her.

'The truth? But isn't it wonderful,' she broke off – 'Mr Chitter has written a weekly article for the past thirty years upon love or hot buttered toast and has sent all his sons to Eton—'

'The truth!' we demanded.

'Oh, the truth,' she stammered, 'the truth has nothing to do with literature,' and sitting down she refused to say another word.

It all seemed to us very inconclusive.

'Ladies, we must try to sum up the results,' Jane was beginning, when a hum, which had been heard for some time through the open window, drowned her voice.

'War! War! War! Declaration of War!' men were shouting in the street below.

We looked at each other in horror.

'What war?' we cried. 'What war?' We remembered, too late, that we had never thought of sending anyone to the House of Commons. We had forgotten all about it. We turned to Poll, who had reached the history shelves in the London Library, and asked her to enlighten us.

'Why,' we cried, 'do men go to war?'

'Sometimes for one reason, sometimes for another,' she replied calmly. 'In 1760, for example—' The shouts outside drowned her words. 'Again in 1797 – in 1804 – It was the Austrians in 1866 – 1870 was the Franco-Prussian – In 1900 on the other hand—'

'But it's now 1914!' we cut her short.

'Ah, I don't know what they're going to war for now,' she admitted.

The war was over and peace was in process of being signed, when I once more found myself with Castalia in the room where our meetings used to be held. We began idly turning over the pages of our old minute books. 'Queer,' I mused, 'to see what we were thinking five years ago.' 'We are agreed,' Castalia quoted, reading over my shoulder, 'that it is the object of life to produce good people and good books.' We made no comment upon *that*. 'A good man is at any rate honest, passionate and unworldly.' 'What a woman's language!' I observed. 'Oh, dear,' cried Castalia, pushing the book away from her, 'what fools we were! It was all Poll's father's fault,' she went on. 'I believe he did it on purpose – that ridiculous will, I mean, forcing Poll to read all the books in the London Library. If we hadn't learnt to read,' she said bitterly, 'we might still have been bearing children in ignorance and that I believe was the happiest life after all. I know what you're going to say about war,' she checked me, 'and the horror of bearing children to see them killed, but our mothers did it, and their mothers, and their mothers before them. And *they* didn't complain. They couldn't read. I've done my best,' she sighed, 'to prevent my little girl from learning to read, but what's the use? I caught Ann only yesterday with a newspaper in her hand and she was beginning to ask me if it was "true". Next she'll ask me whether Mr Lloyd George is a good man, then whether Mr Arnold Bennett is a good novelist, and finally whether I believe in God. How can I bring my daughter up to believe in nothing?' she demanded.

'Surely you could teach her to believe that a man's intellect is, and always will be, fundamentally superior to a woman's?' I suggested. She brightened at this and began to turn over our old minutes again. 'Yes,' she said, 'think of their discoveries, their mathematics, their science, their philosophy, their scholarship—' and then she began to laugh, 'I shall never forget old Hobkin and the hairpin,' she said, and went on reading and laughing and I thought she was quite happy, when suddenly she drew the book from her and burst out, 'Oh, Cassandra, why do you torment me? Don't you know that our belief in man's intellect is the greatest fallacy of them all?' 'What?' I exclaimed. 'Ask any journalist, schoolmaster, politician or public house keeper in the land and they will all tell you that men are much cleverer than women.' 'As if I doubted it,' she said scornfully. 'How could they help it? Haven't we bred them and fed and kept them in comfort since the beginning of time so that they may be clever even if they're nothing else? It's all our doing!' she cried. 'We insisted upon having intellect and now we've got it. And it's intellect,' she continued, 'that's at the bottom of it. What could be more charming than a boy before he has begun to cultivate his intellect? He is beautiful to look at; he gives himself no airs; he understands the meaning of art and literature instinctively; he goes about enjoying his life and making other people enjoy theirs. Then they teach him to cultivate his intellect. He becomes a barrister, a civil servant, a general, an author, a professor. Every day he goes to an office. Every year he produces a book. He maintains a whole family by the products of his brain – poor devil! Soon he cannot come into a room without making us all feel uncomfortable; he condescends to every woman he meets, and dares not tell the truth even to his own wife; instead of rejoicing our eyes we have to shut them if we are to take him in our arms. True, they console themselves with stars of all shapes, ribbons of all shades and incomes of all sizes – but what is to console us? That we shall be able in ten years' time to spend a week-end at Lahore? Or that the least insect in Japan has a name twice the length of its body? Oh, Cassandra, for Heaven's sake let us devise a method by which men may bear children! It is our only chance. For unless we provide them with some innocent occupation we shall get neither good people nor good books; we shall perish beneath the fruits of their unbridled activity; and not a human being will survive to know that there once was Shakespeare!'

'It is too late,' I replied. 'We cannot provide even for the children that we have.'

'And then you ask me to believe in intellect,' she said.

While we spoke, men were crying hoarsely and wearily in the street, and, listening, we heard that the Treaty of Peace had just been signed. The voices died away. The rain was falling and interfered no doubt with the proper explosion of the fireworks.

'My cook will have bought the *Evening News*,' said Castalia, 'and Ann will be spelling it out over her tea. I must go home.'

'It's no good – not a bit of good,' I said. 'Once she knows how to read there's only one thing you can teach her to believe in – and that is herself.'

'Well, that would be a change,' sighed Castalia.

So we swept up the papers of our Society, and, though Ann was playing with her doll very happily, we solemnly made her a present of the lot and told her we had chosen her to be President of the Society of the future – upon which she burst into tears, poor little girl.

THE OTHER TWO

Edith Wharton

I

Waythorn, on the drawing-room hearth, waited for his wife to come down to dinner.

It was their first night under his own roof, and he was surprised at his thrill of boyish agitation. He was not so old, to be sure – his glass gave him little more than the five-and-thirty years to which his wife confessed – but he had fancied himself already in the temperate zone; yet here he was listening for her step with a tender sense of all it symbolized, with some old trail of verse about the garlanded nuptial door-posts floating through his enjoyment of the pleasant room and the good dinner just beyond it.

They had been hastily recalled from their honeymoon by the illness of Lily Haskett, the child of Mrs Waythorn's first marriage. The little girl, at Waythorn's desire, had been transferred to his house on the day of her mother's wedding, and the doctor, on their arrival, broke the news that she was ill with typhoid, but declared that all the symptoms were favourable. Lily could show twelve years of unblemished health, and the case promised to be a light one. The nurse spoke as reassuringly, and after a moment of alarm Mrs Waythorn had adjusted herself to the situation. She was very fond of Lily – her affection for the child had perhaps been her decisive charm in Waythorn's eyes – but she had the perfectly balanced nerves which her little girl had inherited, and no woman ever wasted less tissue in unproductive worry. Waythorn was therefore quite prepared to see her come in presently, a little late because of a last look at Lily, but as serene and well-appointed as if her good-night kiss had been laid on the brow of health. Her composure was restful to him; it acted as ballast to his somewhat unstable sensibilities. As he pictured her bending over the child's bed he thought how soothing her presence must be in illness: her very step would prognosticate recovery.

His own life had been a grey one, from temperament rather than circumstance, and he had been drawn to her by the unperturbed gayety which kept her fresh and elastic at an age when most women's activities are growing either slack or febrile. He knew what was said about her; for, popular as she was, there had always been a faint undercurrent of detraction. When she had appeared in New York, nine or ten years earlier, as the pretty Mrs Haskett whom Gus Varick had unearthed somewhere – was it in Pittsburgh or Utica? – society, while promptly accepting her, had reserved the right to cast a doubt on its own discrimination. Inquiry, however, established her undoubted connection with a socially reigning family, and explained her recent divorce as the natural result of a runaway match at seventeen; and as nothing was known of Mr Haskett it was easy to believe the worst of him.

Alice Haskett's remarriage with Gus Varick was a passport to the set whose recognition she coveted, and for a few years the Varicks were the most popular couple in town. Unfortunately the alliance was brief and stormy, and this time the husband had his champions. Still, even Varick's stanchest supporters admitted that he was not meant for matrimony, and Mrs Varick's grievances were of a nature to bear the inspection of the New York courts. A

New York divorce is in itself a diploma of virtue, and in the semi-widowhood of this second separation Mrs Varick took on an air of sanctity, and was allowed to confide her wrongs to some of the most scrupulous ears in town. But when it was known that she was to marry Waythorn there was a momentary reaction. Her best friends would have preferred to see her remain in the role of the injured wife, which was as becoming to her as crape to a rosy complexion. True, a decent time had elapsed, and it was not even suggested that Waythorn had supplanted his predecessor. Still, people shook their heads over him, and one grudging friend, to whom he affirmed that he took the step with his eyes open, replied oracularly: 'Yes – and with your ears shut.'

Waythorn could afford to smile at these innuendoes. In the Wall Street phrase, he had 'discounted' them. He knew that society has not yet adapted itself to the consequences of divorce, and that till the adaptation takes place every woman who uses the freedom the law accords her must be her own social justification. Waythorn had an amused confidence in his wife's ability to justify herself. His expectations were fulfilled, and before the wedding took place Alice Varick's group had rallied openly to her support. She took it all imperturbably: she had a way of surmounting obstacles without seeming to be aware of them, and Waythorn looked back with wonder at the trivialities over which he had worn his nerves thin. He had the sense of having found refuge in a richer, warmer nature than his own, and his satisfaction, at the moment, was humorously summed up in the thought that his wife, when she had done all she could for Lily, would not be ashamed to come down and enjoy a good dinner.

The anticipation of such enjoyment was not, however, the sentiment expressed by Mrs Waythorn's charming face when she presently joined him. Though she had put on her most engaging teagown she had neglected to assume the smile that went with it, and Waythorn thought he had never seen her look so nearly worried.

'What is it?' he asked. 'Is anything wrong with Lily?'

'No; I've just been in and she's still sleeping.' Mrs Waythorn hesitated. 'But something tiresome has happened.'

He had taken her two hands, and now perceived that he was crushing a paper between them.

'This letter?'

'Yes – Mr Haskett has written – I mean his lawyer has written.'

Waythorn felt himself flush uncomfortably. He dropped his wife's hands.

'What about?'

'About seeing Lily. You know the courts—'

'Yes, yes,' he interrupted nervously.

Nothing was known about Haskett in New York. He was vaguely supposed to have remained in the outer darkness from which his wife had been rescued, and Waythorn was one of the few who were aware that he had given up his business in Utica and followed her to New York in order to be near his little girl. In the days of his wooing, Waythorn had often met Lily on the doorstep, rosy and smiling, on her way 'to see papa'.

'I am so sorry,' Mrs Waythorn murmured.

He roused himself. 'What does he want?'

'He wants to see her. You know she goes to him once a week.'

'Well – he doesn't expect her to go to him now, does he?'

'No – he has heard of her illness; but he expects to come here.'

'Here?'

Mrs Waythorn reddened under his gaze. They looked away from each other.

'I'm afraid he has the right . . . You'll see . . .' She made a proffer of the letter.

Waythorn moved away with a gesture of refusal. He stood staring about the softly lighted room, which a moment before had seemed so full of bridal intimacy.

'I'm so sorry,' she repeated. 'If Lily could have been moved—'

'That's out of the question,' he returned impatiently.

'I suppose so.'

Her lip was beginning to tremble, and he felt himself a brute.

'He must come, of course,' he said. 'When is – his day?'

'I'm afraid – to-morrow.'

'Very well. Send a note in the morning.'

The butler entered to announce dinner.

Waythorn turned to his wife. 'Come – you must be tired. It's beastly, but try to forget about it,' he said, drawing her hand through his arm.

'You're so good, dear. I'll try,' she whispered back.

Her face cleared at once, and as she looked at him across the flowers, between the rosy candle-shades, he saw her lips waver back into a smile.

'How pretty everything is!' she sighed luxuriously.

He turned to the butler. 'The champagne at once, please. Mrs Waythorn is tired.'

In a moment or two their eyes met above the sparkling glasses. Her own were quite clear and untroubled: he saw that she had obeyed his injunction and forgotten.

II

Waythorn, the next morning, went down town earlier than usual. Haskett was not likely to come till the afternoon, but the instinct of flight drove him forth. He meant to stay away all day – he had thoughts of dining at his club. As his door closed behind him he reflected that before he opened it again it would have admitted another man who had as much right to enter it as himself, and the thought filled him with a physical repugnance.

He caught the 'elevated' at the employees' hour, and found himself crushed between two layers of pendulous humanity. At Eighth Street the man facing him wriggled out and another took his place. Waythorn glanced up and saw that it was Gus Varick. The men were so close together that it was impossible to ignore the smile of recognition on Varick's handsome overblown face. And after all – why not? They had always been on good terms, and Varick had been divorced before Waythorn's attentions to his wife began. The two exchanged a word on the perennial grievance of the congested trains, and when a seat at their side was miraculously left empty the instinct of self-preservation made Waythorn slip into it after Varick.

The latter drew the stout man's breath of relief.

'Lord – I was beginning to feel like a pressed flower.' He leaned back, looking unconcernedly at Waythorn. 'Sorry to hear that Sellers is knocked out again.'

'Sellers?' echoed Waythorn, starting at his partner's name.

Varick looked surprised. 'You didn't know he was laid up with the gout?'

'No. I've been away – I only got back last night.' Waythorn felt himself reddening in anticipation of the other's smile.

'Ah – yes; to be sure. And Sellers's attack came on two days ago. I'm afraid he's pretty bad. Very awkward for me, as it happens, because he was just putting through a rather important thing for me.'

'Ah?' Waythorn wondered vaguely since when Varick had been dealing in 'important things'. Hitherto he had dabbled only in the shallow pools of speculation, with which Waythorn's office did not usually concern itself.

It occurred to him that Varick might be talking at random, to relieve the strain of their propinquity. That strain was becoming momentarily more apparent to Waythorn, and when, at Cortlandt Street, he caught sight of an acquaintance, and had a sudden vision of the picture he and Varick must present to an initiated eye, he jumped up with a muttered excuse.

'I hope you'll find Sellers better,' said Varick civilly, and he stammered back: 'If I can be of any use to you—' and let the departing crowd sweep him to the platform.

At his office he heard that Sellers was in fact ill with the gout, and would probably not be able to leave the house for some weeks.

'I'm sorry it should have happened so, Mr Waythorn,' the senior clerk said with affable significance. 'Mr Sellers was very much upset at the idea of giving you such a lot of extra work just now.'

'Oh, that's no matter,' said Waythorn hastily. He secretly welcomed the pressure of additional business, and was glad to think that, when the day's work was over, he would have to call at his partner's on the way home.

He was late for luncheon, and turned in at the nearest restaurant instead of going to his club. The place was full, and the waiter hurried him to the back of the room to capture the only vacant table. In the cloud of cigar-smoke Waythorn did not at once distinguish his neighbours; but presently, looking about him, he saw Varick seated a few feet off. This time, luckily, they were too far apart for conversation, and Varick, who faced another way, had probably not even seen him; but there was an irony in their renewed nearness.

Varick was said to be fond of good living, and as Waythorn sat despatching his hurried luncheon he looked across half enviously at the other's leisurely degustation of his meal. When Waythorn first saw him he had been helping himself with critical deliberation to a bit of Camembert at the ideal point of liquefaction, and now, the cheese removed, he was just pouring his cafe double from its little two-storied earthen pot. He poured slowly, his ruddy profile bent above the task, and one beringed white hand steadying the lid of the coffee-pot; then he stretched his other hand to the decanter of cognac at his elbow, filled a liqueur-glass, took a tentative sip and poured the brandy into his coffee-cup.

Waythorn watched him in a kind of fascination. What was he thinking of – only of the flavour of the coffee and the liqueur? Had the morning's meeting left no more trace in his thoughts than on his face? Had his wife so completely passed out of his life that even this odd encounter with her present husband, within a week after her remarriage, was no more than an incident in his day? And as Waythorn mused, another idea struck him: had Haskett ever met Varick as Varick and he had just met? The recollection of Haskett perturbed him, and he rose and left the restaurant, taking a circuitous way out to escape the placid irony of Varick's nod.

It was after seven when Waythorn reached home. He thought the footman who opened the door looked at him oddly.

'How is Miss Lily?' he asked in haste.

'Doing very well, sir. A gentleman—'

'Tell Barlow to put off dinner for half an hour,' Waythorn cut him off, hurrying upstairs.

He went straight to his room and dressed without seeing his wife. When he reached the drawing-room she was there, fresh and radiant. Lily's day had been good; the doctor was not coming back that evening.

At dinner Waythorn told her of Sellers's illness and of the resulting complications. She listened sympathetically, adjuring him not to let himself be overworked, and asking vague feminine questions about the routine of the office. Then she gave him the chronicle of Lily's day; quoted the nurse and doctor, and told him who had called to inquire. He had never seen her more serene and unruffled. It struck him, with a curious pang, that she was very happy in being with him, so happy that she found a childish pleasure in rehearsing the trivial incidents of her day.

After dinner they went to the library, and the servant put the coffee and liqueurs on a low table before her and left the room. She looked singularly soft and girlish in her rosy pale dress, against the dark leather of one of his bachelor armchairs. A day earlier the contrast would have charmed him.

He turned away now, choosing a cigar with affected deliberation. 'Did Haskett come?' he asked, with his back to her.

'Oh, yes – he came.'

'You didn't see him, of course?'

She hesitated a moment. 'I let the nurse see him.'

That was all. There was nothing more to ask. He swung round toward her, applying a match to his cigar. Well, the thing was over for a week, at any rate. He would try not to think of it. She looked up at him, a trifle rosier than usual, with a smile in her eyes.

'Ready for your coffee, dear?'

He leaned against the mantelpiece, watching her as she lifted the coffee-pot. The lamplight struck a gleam from her bracelets and tipped her soft hair with brightness. How light and slender she was, and how each gesture flowed into the next! She seemed a creature all compact of harmonies. As the thought of Haskett receded, Waythorn felt himself yielding again to the joy of possessorship. They were his, those white hands with their flitting motions, his the light haze of hair, the lips and eyes . . .

She set down the coffee-pot, and reaching for the decanter of cognac, measured off a liqueur-glass and poured it into his cup.

Waythorn uttered a sudden exclamation.

'What is the matter?' she said, startled.

'Nothing; only – I don't take cognac in my coffee.'

'Oh, how stupid of me,' she cried.

Their eyes met, and she blushed a sudden agonized red.

III

Ten days later, Mr Sellers, still house-bound, asked Waythorn to call on his way down town.

The senior partner, with his swaddled foot propped up by the fire, greeted his associate with an air of embarrassment.

'I'm sorry, my dear fellow; I've got to ask you to do an awkward thing for me.'

Waythorn waited, and the other went on, after a pause apparently given to the arrangement of his phrases: 'The fact is, when I was knocked out I had just gone into a rather complicated piece of business for – Gus Varick.'

'Well?' said Waythorn, with an attempt to put him at his ease.

'Well – it's this way: Varick came to me the day before my attack. He had evidently had an inside tip from somebody, and had made about a hundred thousand. He came to me for advice, and I suggested his going in with Vanderlyn.'

'Oh, the deuce!' Waythorn exclaimed. He saw in a flash what had happened. The investment was an alluring one, but required negotiation. He listened intently while Sellers put the case before him, and, the statement ended, he said: 'You think I ought to see Varick?'

'I'm afraid I can't as yet. The doctor is obdurate. And this thing can't wait. I hate to ask you, but no one else in the office knows the ins and outs of it.'

Waythorn stood silent. He did not care a farthing for the success of Varick's venture, but the honour of the office was to be considered, and he could hardly refuse to oblige his partner.

'Very well,' he said, 'I'll do it.'

That afternoon, apprised by telephone, Varick called at the

office. Waythorn, waiting in his private room, wondered what the others thought of it. The newspapers, at the time of Mrs Waythorn's marriage, had acquainted their readers with every detail of her previous matrimonial ventures, and Waythorn could fancy the clerks smiling behind Varick's back as he was ushered in.

Varick bore himself admirably. He was easy without being undignified, and Waythorn was conscious of cutting a much less impressive figure. Varick had no head for business, and the talk prolonged itself for nearly an hour while Waythorn set forth with scrupulous precision the details of the proposed transaction.

'I'm awfully obliged to you,' Varick said as he rose. 'The fact is I'm not used to having much money to look after, and I don't want to make an ass of myself—' He smiled, and Waythorn could not help noticing that there was something pleasant about his smile. 'It feels uncommonly queer to have enough cash to pay one's bills. I'd have sold my soul for it a few years ago!'

Waythorn winced at the allusion. He had heard it rumoured that a lack of funds had been one of the determining causes of the Varick separation, but it did not occur to him that Varick's words were intentional. It seemed more likely that the desire to keep clear of embarrassing topics had fatally drawn him into one. Waythorn did not wish to be outdone in civility.

'We'll do the best we can for you,' he said. 'I think this is a good thing you're in.'

'Oh, I'm sure it's immense. It's awfully good of you—' Varick broke off, embarrassed. 'I suppose the thing's settled now – but if—'

'If anything happens before Sellers is about, I'll see you again,' said Waythorn quietly. He was glad, in the end, to appear the more self-possessed of the two.

The course of Lily's illness ran smooth, and as the days passed Waythorn grew used to the idea of Haskett's weekly visit. The first time the day came round, he stayed out late, and questioned his wife as to the visit on his return. She replied at once that Haskett had merely seen the nurse downstairs, as the doctor did not wish any one in the child's sick-room till after the crisis.

The following week Waythorn was again conscious of the recurrence of the day, but had forgotten it by the time he came home to dinner. The crisis of the disease came a few days later, with a rapid decline of fever, and the little girl was pronounced out of danger. In the rejoicing which ensued the thought of Haskett passed out of Waythorn's mind and one afternoon, letting himself into the house with a latchkey, he went straight to his library without noticing a shabby hat and umbrella in the hall.

In the library he found a small effaced-looking man with a thinnish grey beard sitting on the edge of a chair. The stranger might have been a piano-tuner, or one of those mysteriously efficient persons who are summoned in emergencies to adjust some detail of the domestic machinery. He blinked at Waythorn through a pair of gold-rimmed spectacles and said mildly: 'Mr Waythorn, I presume? I am Lily's father.'

Waythorn flushed. 'Oh—' he stammered uncomfortably. He broke off, disliking to appear rude. Inwardly he was trying to adjust the actual Haskett to the image of him projected by his wife's reminiscences. Waythorn had been allowed to infer that Alice's first husband was a brute.

'I am sorry to intrude,' said Haskett, with his over-the-counter politeness.

'Don't mention it,' returned Waythorn, collecting himself. 'I suppose the nurse has been told?'

'I presume so. I can wait,' said Haskett. He had a resigned way of speaking, as though life had worn down his natural powers of resistance.

Waythorn stood on the threshold, nervously pulling off his gloves.

'I'm sorry you've been detained. I will send for the nurse,' he said; and as he opened the door he added with an effort: 'I'm glad we can give you a good report of Lily.' He winced as the we slipped out, but Haskett seemed not to notice it.

'Thank you, Mr Waythorn. It's been an anxious time for me.'

'Ah, well, that's past. Soon she'll be able to go to you.' Waythorn nodded and passed out.

In his own room, he flung himself down with a groan. He hated the womanish sensibility which made him suffer so acutely from the grotesque chances of life. He had known when he married that his wife's former husbands were both living, and that amid the multiplied contacts of modern existence there were a thousand chances to one that he would run against one or the other, yet he found himself as much disturbed by his brief encounter with Haskett as though the law had not obligingly removed all difficulties in the way of their meeting.

Waythorn sprang up and began to pace the room nervously. He had not suffered half so much from his two meetings with Varick. It was Haskett's presence in his own house that made the situation so intolerable. He stood still, hearing steps in the passage.

'This way, please,' he heard the nurse say. Haskett was being taken upstairs, then: not a corner of the house but was open to him. Waythorn dropped into another chair, staring vaguely ahead of him. On his dressing-table stood a photograph of Alice, taken when he had first known her. She was Alice Varick then – how fine and exquisite he had thought her! Those were Varick's pearls about her neck. At Waythorn's instance they had been returned before her marriage. Had Haskett ever given her any trinkets – and what had become of them, Waythorn wondered? He realized suddenly that he knew very little of Haskett's past or present situation; but from the man's appearance and manner of speech he could reconstruct with curious precision the surroundings of Alice's first marriage. And it startled him to think that she had, in the background of her life, a phase of existence so different from anything with which he had connected her. Varick, whatever his faults, was a gentleman, in the conventional, traditional sense of the term: the sense which at that moment seemed, oddly enough, to have most meaning to Waythorn. He and Varick had the same social habits, spoke the same language, understood the same allusions. But this other man . . . it was grotesquely uppermost in Waythorn's mind that Haskett had worn a made-up tie attached with an elastic. Why should that ridiculous detail symbolize the whole man? Waythorn was exasperated by his own paltriness, but the fact of the tie expanded, forced itself on him, became as it were the key to Alice's past. He could see her, as Mrs Haskett, sitting in a 'front parlour' furnished in plush, with a pianola, and a copy of 'Ben Hur' on the centre-table. He could see her going to the theatre with Haskett – or perhaps even to a 'Church Sociable' – she in a 'picture hat' and Haskett in a black frock-coat, a little creased, with the made-up tie on an elastic. On the way home they would stop and look at the illuminated shop-windows, lingering over the photographs of New York actresses. On Sunday afternoons Haskett would take her for a walk, pushing Lily ahead of them in a white enamelled perambulator, and Waythorn had a vision of the people they would stop and talk to. He could fancy how pretty Alice must have looked, in a dress adroitly constructed from the hints of a New York fashion-paper; how she must have looked down on the other women, chafing at her life, and secretly feeling that she belonged in a bigger place.

For the moment his foremost thought was one of wonder at

the way in which she had shed the phase of existence which her marriage with Haskett implied. It was as if her whole aspect, every gesture, every inflection, every allusion, were a studied negation of that period of her life. If she had denied being married to Haskett she could hardly have stood more convicted of duplicity than in this obliteration of the self which had been his wife.

Waythorn started up, checking himself in the analysis of her motives. What right had he to create a fantastic effigy of her and then pass judgment on it? She had spoken vaguely of her first marriage as unhappy, had hinted, with becoming reticence, that Haskett had wrought havoc among her young illusions . . . It was a pity for Waythorn's peace of mind that Haskett's very inoffensiveness shed a new light on the nature of those illusions. A man would rather think that his wife has been brutalized by her first husband than that the process has been reversed.

'Why, how do you do?' she said with a distinct note of pleasure.

IV

'Mr Waythorn, I don't like that French governess of Lily's.'

Haskett, subdued and apologetic, stood before Waythorn in the library, revolving his shabby hat in his hand.

Waythorn, surprised in his armchair over the evening paper, stared back perplexedly at his visitor.

'You'll excuse my asking to see you,' Haskett continued. 'But this is my last visit, and I thought if I could have a word with you it would be a better way than writing to Mrs Waythorn's lawyer.'

Waythorn rose uneasily. He did not like the French governess either; but that was irrelevant.

'I am not so sure of that,' he returned stiffly; 'but since you wish it I will give your message to – my wife.' He always hesitated over the possessive pronoun in addressing Haskett.

The latter sighed. 'I don't know as that will help much. She didn't like it when I spoke to her.'

Waythorn turned red. 'When did you see her?' he asked.

'Not since the first day I came to see Lily – right after she was taken sick. I remarked to her then that I didn't like the governess.'

Waythorn made no answer. He remembered distinctly that, after that first visit, he had asked his wife if she had seen Haskett. She had lied to him then, but she had respected his wishes since; and the incident cast a curious light on her character. He was sure she would not have seen Haskett that first day if she had divined that Waythorn would object, and the fact that she did not divine it was almost as disagreeable to the latter as the discovery that she had lied to him.

'I don't like the woman,' Haskett was repeating with mild persistency. 'She ain't straight, Mr Waythorn – she'll teach the child to be underhand. I've noticed a change in Lily – she's too anxious to please – and she don't always tell the truth. She used to be the straightest child, Mr Waythorn—' He broke off, his voice a little thick. 'Not but what I want her to have a stylish education,' he ended.

Waythorn was touched. 'I'm sorry, Mr Haskett; but frankly, I don't quite see what I can do.'

Haskett hesitated. Then he laid his hat on the table, and advanced to the hearth-rug, on which Waythorn was standing. There was nothing aggressive in his manner; but he had the solemnity of a timid man resolved on a decisive measure.

'There's just one thing you can do, Mr Waythorn,' he said. 'You can remind Mrs Waythorn that, by the decree of the courts, I am entitled to have a voice in Lily's bringing up.' He paused, and went on more deprecatingly: 'I'm not the kind to talk about enforcing my rights, Mr Waythorn. I don't know as I think a man is entitled to rights he hasn't known how to hold on to; but this business of the child is different. I've never let go there – and I never mean to.'

The scene left Waythorn deeply shaken. Shamefacedly, in indirect ways, he had been finding out about Haskett; and all that he had learned was favourable. The little man, in order to be near his daughter, had sold out his share in a profitable business in Utica, and accepted a modest clerkship in a New York manufacturing house. He boarded in a shabby street and had few acquaintances. His passion for Lily filled his life. Waythorn felt that this exploration of Haskett was like groping about with a dark-lantern in his wife's past; but he saw now that there were recesses his lantern had not explored. He had never inquired into the exact circumstances of his wife's first matrimonial rupture. On the surface all had been fair. It was she who had obtained the divorce, and the court had given her the child. But Waythorn knew how many ambiguities such a verdict might cover. The mere fact that Haskett retained a right over his daughter implied an unsuspected compromise. Waythorn was an idealist. He always refused to recognize unpleasant contingencies till he found himself confronted with them, and then he saw them followed by a special train of consequences. His next days were thus haunted, and he determined to try to lay the ghosts by conjuring them up in his wife's presence.

When he repeated Haskett's request a flame of anger passed over her face; but she subdued it instantly and spoke with a slight quiver of outraged motherhood.

'It is very ungentlemanly of him,' she said.

The word grated on Waythorn. 'That is neither here nor there. It's a bare question of rights.'

She murmured: 'It's not as if he could ever be a help to Lily—'

Waythorn flushed. This was even less to his taste. 'The question is,' he repeated, 'what authority has he over her?'

She looked downward, twisting herself a little in her seat. 'I am willing to see him – I thought you objected,' she faltered.

In a flash he understood that she knew the extent of Haskett's claims. Perhaps it was not the first time she had resisted them.

'My objecting has nothing to do with it,' he said coldly; 'if Haskett has a right to be consulted you must consult him.'

She burst into tears, and he saw that she expected him to regard her as a victim.

Haskett did not abuse his rights. Waythorn had felt miserably sure that he would not. But the governess was dismissed, and from time to time the little man demanded an interview with Alice. After the first outburst she accepted the situation with her usual adaptability. Haskett had once reminded Waythorn of the piano-tuner, and Mrs Waythorn, after a month or two, appeared to class him with that domestic familiar. Waythorn could not but respect the father's tenacity. At first he had tried to cultivate the suspicion that Haskett might be 'up to' something, that he had an object in securing a foothold in the house. But in his heart Waythorn was sure of Haskett's single-mindedness; he even guessed in the latter a mild contempt for such advantages as his relation with the Waythorns might offer. Haskett's sincerity of purpose made him invulnerable, and his successor had to accept him as a lien on the property.

Mr Sellers was sent to Europe to recover from his gout, and Varick's affairs hung on Waythorn's hands. The negotiations were prolonged and complicated; they necessitated frequent conferences between the two men, and the interests of the firm forbade Waythorn's suggesting that his client should transfer his business to another office.

Varick appeared well in the transaction. In moments of relaxation his coarse streak appeared, and Waythorn dreaded his geniality; but in the office he was concise and clear-headed, with a flattering deference to Waythorn's judgment. Their business relations being so affably established, it would have been absurd for the two men to ignore each other in society. The first time they met in a drawing-room, Varick took up their intercourse in the same easy key, and his hostess's grateful glance obliged Waythorn to respond to it. After that they ran across each other frequently, and one evening at a ball Waythorn, wandering through the remoter rooms, came upon Varick seated beside his wife. She coloured a little, and faltered in what she was saying; but Varick nodded to Waythorn without rising, and the latter strolled on.

In the carriage, on the way home, he broke out nervously: 'I didn't know you spoke to Varick.'

Her voice trembled a little. 'It's the first time – he happened to be standing near me; I didn't know what to do. It's so awkward, meeting everywhere – and he said you had been very kind about some business.'

'That's different,' said Waythorn.

She paused a moment. 'I'll do just as you wish,' she returned pliantly. 'I thought it would be less awkward to speak to him when we meet.'

Her pliancy was beginning to sicken him. Had she really no will of her own – no theory about her relation to these men? She had accepted Haskett – did she mean to accept Varick? It was 'less awkward', as she had said, and her instinct was to evade difficulties or to circumvent them. With sudden vividness Waythorn saw how the instinct had developed. She was 'as easy as an old shoe' – a shoe that too many feet had worn. Her elasticity was the result of tension in too many different directions. Alice Haskett – Alice Varick – Alice Waythorn – she had been each in turn, and had left hanging to each name a little of her privacy, a little of her personality, a little of the inmost self where the unknown god abides.

'Yes – it's better to speak to Varick,' said Waythorn wearily.

V

The winter wore on, and society took advantage of the Waythorns' acceptance of Varick. Harassed hostesses were grateful to them for bridging over a social difficulty, and Mrs Waythorn was held up as a miracle of good taste. Some experimental spirits could not resist the diversion of throwing Varick and his former wife together, and there were those who thought he found a zest in the propinquity. But Mrs Waythorn's conduct remained irreproachable. She neither avoided Varick nor sought him out. Even Waythorn could not but admit that she had discovered the solution of the newest social problem.

He had married her without giving much thought to that problem. He had fancied that a woman can shed her past like a man. But now he saw that Alice was bound to hers both by the circumstances which forced her into continued relation with it, and by the traces it had left on her nature. With grim irony Waythorn compared himself to a member of a syndicate. He held so many shares in his wife's personality and his predecessors were his partners in the business. If there had been any element of passion in the transaction he would have felt less deteriorated by it. The fact that Alice took her change of husbands like a change of weather reduced the situation to mediocrity. He could have forgiven her for blunders, for excesses; for resisting Hackett, for yielding to Varick; for anything but her acquiescence and her tact. She reminded him of a juggler tossing knives; but the knives were blunt and she knew they would never cut her.

And then, gradually, habit formed a protecting surface for his sensibilities. If he paid for each day's comfort with the small change of his illusions, he grew daily to value the comfort more and set less store upon the coin. He had drifted into a dulling propinquity with Haskett and Varick and he took refuge in the cheap revenge of satirizing the situation. He even began to reckon up the advantages which accrued from it, to ask himself if it were not better to own a third of a wife who knew how to make a man happy than a whole one who had lacked opportunity to acquire the art. For it was an art, and made up, like all others, of concessions, eliminations and embellishments; of lights judiciously thrown and shadows skilfully softened. His wife knew exactly how to manage the lights, and he knew exactly to what training she owed her skill. He even tried to trace the source of his obligations, to discriminate between the influences which had combined to produce his domestic happiness: he perceived that Haskett's commonness had made Alice worship good breeding, while Varick's liberal construction of the marriage bond had taught her to value the conjugal virtues; so that he was directly indebted to his predecessors for the devotion which made his life easy if not inspiring.

From this phase he passed into that of complete acceptance. He ceased to satirize himself because time dulled the irony of the situation and the joke lost its humour with its sting. Even the sight of Haskett's hat on the hall table had ceased to touch the springs of epigram. The hat was often seen there now, for it had been decided that it was better for Lily's father to visit her than for the little girl to go to his boarding-house. Waythorn, having acquiesced in this arrangement, had been surprised to find how little difference it made. Haskett was never obtrusive, and the few visitors who met him on the stairs were unaware of his identity. Waythorn did not know how often he saw Alice, but with himself Haskett was seldom in contact.

One afternoon, however, he learned on entering that Lily's father was waiting to see him. In the library he found Haskett occupying a chair in his usual provisional way. Waythorn always felt grateful to him for not leaning back.

'I hope you'll excuse me, Mr Waythorn,' he said rising. 'I wanted to see Mrs Waythorn about Lily, and your man asked me to wait here till she came in.'

'Of course,' said Waythorn, remembering that a sudden leak had that morning given over the drawing-room to the plumbers.

He opened his cigar-case and held it out to his visitor, and Haskett's acceptance seemed to mark a fresh stage in their intercourse. The spring evening was chilly, and Waythorn invited his guest to draw up his chair to the fire. He meant to find an excuse to leave Haskett in a moment; but he was tired and cold, and after all the little man no longer jarred on him.

The two were inclosed in the intimacy of their blended cigar-smoke when the door opened and Varick walked into the room. Waythorn rose abruptly. It was the first time that Varick had come to the house, and the surprise of seeing him, combined with the singular inopportuneness of his arrival, gave a new edge to Waythorn's blunted sensibilities. He stared at his visitor without speaking.

Varick seemed too preoccupied to notice his host's embarrassment.

'My dear fellow,' he exclaimed in his most expansive tone, 'I must apologize for tumbling in on you in this way, but I was too late to catch you down town, and so I thought—' He stopped short, catching sight of Haskett, and his sanguine colour deepened to a flush which spread vividly under his scant blond hair. But in a moment he recovered himself and nodded slightly. Haskett returned the bow in silence, and Waythorn was still groping for speech when the footman came in carrying a tea-table.

The intrusion offered a welcome vent to Waythorn's nerves. 'What the deuce are you bringing this here for?' he said sharply.

'I beg your pardon, sir, but the plumbers are still in the drawing-room, and Mrs Waythorn said she would have tea in the library.' The footman's perfectly respectful tone implied a reflection on Waythorn's reasonableness.

'Oh, very well,' said the latter resignedly, and the footman proceeded to open the folding tea-table and set out its complicated appointments. While this interminable process continued the three men stood motionless, watching it with a fascinated stare, till Waythorn, to break the silence, said to Varick: 'Won't you have a cigar?'

He held out the case he had just tendered to Haskett, and Varick helped himself with a smile. Waythorn looked about for a match, and finding none, proffered a light from his own cigar. Haskett, in the background, held his ground mildly, examining his cigar-tip now and then, and stepping forward at the right moment to knock its ashes into the fire.

The footman at last withdrew, and Varick immediately began: 'If I could just say half a word to you about this business—'

'Certainly,' stammered Waythorn; 'in the dining-room—'

But as he placed his hand on the door it opened from without, and his wife appeared on the threshold.

She came in fresh and smiling, in her street dress and hat, shedding a fragrance from the boa which she loosened in advancing.

'Shall we have tea in here, dear?' she began; and then she caught sight of Varick. Her smile deepened, veiling a slight tremor of surprise. 'Why, how do you do?' she said with a distinct note of pleasure.

As she shook hands with Varick she saw Haskett standing behind him. Her smile faded for a moment, but she recalled it quickly, with a scarcely perceptible side-glance at Waythorn.

'How do you do, Mr Haskett?' she said, and shook hands with him a shade less cordially.

The three men stood awkwardly before her, till Varick, always the most self-possessed, dashed into an explanatory phrase.

'We – I had to see Waythorn a moment on business,' he stammered, brick-red from chin to nape.

Haskett stepped forward with his air of mild obstinacy. 'I am sorry to intrude; but you appointed five o'clock—' he directed his resigned glance to the time-piece on the mantel.

She swept aside their embarrassment with a charming gesture of hospitality.

'I'm so sorry – I'm always late; but the afternoon was so lovely.' She stood drawing her gloves off, propitiatory and graceful, diffusing about her a sense of ease and familiarity in which the situation lost its grotesqueness. 'But before talking business,' she added brightly, 'I'm sure every one wants a cup of tea.'

She dropped into her low chair by the tea-table, and the two visitors, as if drawn by her smile, advanced to receive the cups she held out.

She glanced about for Waythorn, and he took the third cup with a laugh.

AN EXCERPT FROM
PRIDE AND PREJUDICE

Jane Austen

CHAPTER I

It is a truth universally acknowledged, that a single man in possession of a good fortune, must be in want of a wife.

However little known the feelings or views of such a man may be on his first entering a neighbourhood, this truth is so well fixed in the minds of the surrounding families, that he is considered as the rightful property of some one or other of their daughters.

'My dear Mr Bennet,' said his lady to him one day, 'have you heard that Netherfield Park is let at last?'

Mr Bennet replied that he had not.

'But it is,' returned she; 'for Mrs Long has just been here, and she told me all about it.'

Mr Bennet made no answer.

'Do not you want to know who has taken it?' cried his wife impatiently.

'*You* want to tell me, and I have no objection to hearing it.'

This was invitation enough.

'Why, my dear, you must know, Mrs Long says that Netherfield is taken by a young man of large fortune from the north of England; that he came down on Monday in a chaise and four to see the place, and was so much delighted with it that he agreed with Mr Morris immediately; that he is to take possession before Michaelmas, and some of his servants are to be in the house by the end of next week.'

'What is his name?'

'Bingley.'

'Is he married or single?'

'Oh! single, my dear, to be sure! A single man of large fortune; four or five thousand a year. What a fine thing for our girls!'

'How so? how can it affect them?'

'My dear Mr Bennet,' replied his wife, 'how can you be so tiresome! You must know that I am thinking of his marrying one of them.'

'Is that his design in settling here?'

'Design! nonsense, how can you talk so! But it is very likely that he may fall in love with one of them, and therefore you must visit him as soon as he comes.'

'I see no occasion for that. You and the girls may go, or you may send them by themselves, which perhaps will be still better, for as you are as handsome as any of them, Mr Bingley might like you the best of the party.'

'My dear, you flatter me. I certainly *have* had my share of beauty, but I do not pretend to be any thing extraordinary now. When a woman has five grown up daughters, she ought to give over thinking of her own beauty.'

'In such cases, a woman has not often much beauty to think of.'

'But, my dear, you must indeed go and see Mr Bingley when he comes into the neighbourhood.'

'It is more than I engage for, I assure you.'

'But consider your daughters. Only think what an establishment it would be for one of them. Sir William and Lady Lucas are determined to go, merely on that account, for in general you know they visit no new comers. Indeed you must go, for it will be impossible for *us* to visit him, if you do not.'

'You are over scrupulous surely. I dare say Mr Bingley will be very glad to see you; and I will send a few lines by you to assure him of my hearty consent to his marrying which ever he chuses of the girls; though I must throw in a good word for my little Lizzy.'

'I desire you will do no such thing. Lizzy is not a bit better than the others; and I am sure she is not half so handsome as Jane, nor half so good humoured as Lydia. But you are always giving *her* the preference.'

'They have none of them much to recommend them,' replied he; 'they are all silly and ignorant like other girls; but Lizzy has something more of quickness than her sisters.'

'Mr Bennet, how can you abuse your own children in such a way? You take delight in vexing me. You have no compassion on my poor nerves.'

'You mistake me, my dear. I have a high respect for your nerves. They are my old friends. I have heard you mention them with consideration these twenty years at least.'

'Ah! you do not know what I suffer.'

'But I hope you will get over it, and live to see many young men of four thousand a year come into the neighbourhood.'

'It will be no use to us, if twenty such should come since you will not visit them.'

'Depend upon it, my dear, that when there are twenty, I will visit them all.'

Mr Bennet was so odd a mixture of quick parts, sarcastic humour, reserve and caprice, that the experience of three and twenty years had been insufficient to make his wife understand his character. *Her* mind was less difficult to develope. She was a woman of mean understanding, little information and uncertain temper. When she was discontented she fancied herself nervous. The business of her life was to get her daughters married; its solace was visiting and news.

CHAPTER II

Mr Bennet was among the earliest of those who waited on Mr Bingley. He had always intended to visit him, though to the last always assuring his wife that he should not go; and till the evening after the visit was paid, she had no knowledge of it. It was then disclosed in the following manner. Observing his second daughter employed in trimming a hat, he suddenly addressed her with,

'I hope Mr Bingley will like it, Lizzy.'

'We are not in a way to know *what* Mr Bingley likes,' said her mother resentfully, 'since we are not to visit.'

'But you forget, mama,' said Elizabeth, 'that we shall meet him at the assemblies, and that Mrs Long has promised to introduce him.'

'I do not believe Mrs Long will do any such thing. She has two nieces of her own. She is a selfish, hypocritical woman, and I have no opinion of her.'

'No more have I,' said Mr Bennet; 'and I am glad to find that you do not depend on her serving you.'

Mrs Bennet deigned not to make any reply; but unable to contain herself, began scolding one of her daughters.

'Don't keep coughing so, Kitty, for heaven's sake! Have a little compassion on my nerves. You tear them to pieces.'

'Kitty has no discretion in her coughs,' said her father; 'she times them ill.'

'I do not cough for my own amusement,' replied Kitty fretfully.

'When is your next ball to be, Lizzy?'

'To-morrow fortnight.'

'Aye, so it is,' cried her mother, 'and Mrs Long does not come back till the day before; so, it will be impossible for her to introduce him, for she will not know him herself.'

'Then, my dear, you may have the advantage of your friend, and introduce Mr Bingley to *her*.'

'Impossible, Mr Bennet, impossible, when I am not acquainted with him myself; how can you be so teazing?'

'I honour your circumspection. A fortnight's acquaintance is certainly very little. One cannot know what a man really is by the end of a fortnight. But if we do not venture, somebody else will; and after all, Mrs Long and her nieces must stand their chance; and therefore, as she will think it an act of kindness, if you decline the office, I will take it on myself.'

The girls stared at their father. Mrs Bennet said only, 'Nonsense, nonsense!'

'What can be the meaning of that emphatic exclamation?' cried he. 'Do you consider the forms of introduction, and the stress that is laid on them, as nonsense? I cannot quite agree with you *there*. What say you, Mary? for you are a young lady of deep reflection I know, and read great books, and make extracts.'

Mary wished to say something very sensible, but knew not how.

'While Mary is adjusting her ideas,' he continued, 'let us return to Mr Bingley.'

'I am sick of Mr Bingley,' cried his wife.

'I am sorry to hear *that*; but why did not you tell me so before? If I had known as much this morning, I certainly would not have called on him. It is very unlucky; but as I have actually paid the visit, we cannot escape the acquaintance now.'

The astonishment of the ladies was just what he wished; that of Mrs Bennet perhaps surpassing the rest; though when the first tumult of joy was over, she began to declare that it was what she had expected all the while.

'How good it was in you, my dear Mr Bennet! But I knew I should persuade you at last. I was sure you loved your girls too well to neglect such an acquaintance. Well, how pleased I am! and it is such a good joke, too, that you should have gone this morning, and never said a word about it till now.'

'Now, Kitty, you may cough as much as you chuse,' said Mr Bennet; and, as he spoke, he left the room, fatigued with the raptures of his wife.

'What an excellent father you have, girls,' said she, when the door was shut. 'I do not know how you will ever make him amends for his kindness; or me either, for that matter. At our time of life, it is not so pleasant I can tell you, to be making new acquaintance every day; but for your sakes, we would do any thing. Lydia, my love, though you *are* the youngest, I dare say Mr Bingley will dance with you at the next ball.'

'Oh!' said Lydia stoutly, 'I am not afraid; for though I *am* the youngest, I'm the tallest.'

The rest of the evening was spent in conjecturing how soon he would return Mr Bennet's visit, and determining when they should ask him to dinner.

CHAPTER III

Not all that Mrs Bennet, however, with the assistance of her five daughters, could ask on the subject was sufficient to draw from her husband any satisfactory description of Mr Bingley. They attacked him in various ways; with barefaced questions, ingenious suppositions and distant surmises; but he eluded the skill of them all; and they were at last obliged to accept the second-hand intelligence of their neighbour Lady Lucas. Her report was highly favourable. Sir William had been delighted with him. He was quite young, wonderfully handsome, extremely agreeable and to crown the whole, he meant to be at the next assembly with a large party. Nothing could be more delightful! To be fond of dancing was a certain step towards falling in love; and very lively hopes of Mr Bingley's heart were entertained.

'If I can but see one of my daughters happily settled at Netherfield,' said Mrs Bennet to her husband, 'and all the others equally well married, I shall have nothing to wish for.'

In a few days Mr Bingley returned Mr Bennet's visit, and sat about ten minutes with him in his library. He had entertained hopes of being admitted to a sight of the young ladies, of whose beauty he had heard much; but he saw only the father. The ladies were somewhat more fortunate, for they had the advantage of ascertaining from an upper window, that he wore a blue coat and rode a black horse.

An invitation to dinner was soon afterwards dispatched; and already had Mrs Bennet planned the courses that were to do credit to her housekeeping, when an answer arrived which deferred it all. Mr Bingley was obliged to be in town the following day, and consequently unable to accept the honour of their invitation, &c. Mrs Bennet was quite disconcerted. She could not imagine what business he could have in town so soon after his arrival in Hertfordshire; and she began to fear that he might be always flying about from one place to another, and never settled at Netherfield as he ought to be. Lady Lucas quieted her fears a little by starting the idea of his being gone to London only to get a large party for the ball; and a report soon followed that Mr Bingley was to bring twelve ladies and seven gentlemen with him to the assembly. The girls grieved over such a number of ladies; but were comforted the day before the ball by hearing, that instead of twelve, he had brought only six with him from London, his five sisters and a cousin. And when the party entered the assembly room, it consisted of only five altogether; Mr Bingley, his two sisters, the husband of the eldest and another young man.

Mr Bingley was good looking and gentleman-like; he had a pleasant countenance, and easy, unaffected manners. His sisters were fine women, with an air of decided fashion. His brother-in-law, Mr Hurst, merely looked the gentleman; but his friend Mr Darcy soon drew the attention of the room by his fine, tall person, handsome features, noble mien; and the report which was in general circulation within five minutes after his entrance, of his having ten thousand a year. The gentlemen pronounced him to be a fine figure of a man, the ladies declared he was much handsomer than Mr Bingley, and he was looked at with great admiration for about half the evening, till his manners gave a disgust which turned the tide of his popularity; for he was discovered to be proud, to be above his company and above being pleased; and not all his large estate in Derbyshire could then save him from having a most forbidding, disagreeable countenance, and being unworthy to be compared with his friend.

Mr Bingley had soon made himself acquainted with all the principal people in the room; he was lively and unreserved, danced every dance, was angry that the ball closed so early and talked of giving one himself at Netherfield. Such amiable qualities must speak for themselves. What a contrast between him and his friend! Mr Darcy danced only once with Mrs Hurst and once with Miss Bingley, declined being introduced to any other lady and spent the rest of the evening in walking about the room, speaking occasionally to one of his own party. His character was decided. He was the proudest, most disagreeable man in the world, and every body hoped that he would never come there again. Amongst the most violent against him was Mrs Bennet, whose dislike of his general behaviour, was sharpened into particular resentment, by his having slighted one of her daughters.

Elizabeth Bennet had been obliged, by the scarcity of gentlemen, to sit down for two dances; and during part of that time, Mr Darcy had been standing near enough for her to overhear a conversation between him and Mr Bingley, who came from the dance for a few minutes, to press his friend to join it.

'Come, Darcy,' said he, 'I must have you dance. I hate to see you standing about by yourself in this stupid manner. You had much better dance.'

'I certainly shall not. You know how I detest it, unless I am particularly acquainted with my partner. At such an assembly as this, it would be insupportable. Your sisters are engaged, and there is not another woman in the room, whom it would not be a punishment to me to stand up with.'

'I would not be so fastidious as you are,' cried Bingley, 'for a kingdom! Upon my honour, I never met with so many pleasant girls in my life, as I have this evening; and there are several of them you see uncommonly pretty.'

'*You* are dancing with the only handsome girl in the room,' said Mr Darcy, looking at the eldest Miss Bennet.

'Oh! she is the most beautiful creature I ever beheld! But there is one of her sisters sitting down just behind you, who is very pretty, and I dare say, very agreeable. Do let me ask my partner to introduce you.'

'Which do you mean?' and turning round, he looked for a moment at Elizabeth, till catching her eye, he withdrew his own and coldly said, 'She is tolerable; but not handsome enough to tempt *me*; and I am in no humour at present to give consequence to young ladies who are slighted by other men. You had better return to your partner and enjoy her smiles, for you are wasting your time with me.'

Mr Bingley followed his advice. Mr Darcy walked off; and

Elizabeth remained with no very cordial feelings towards him. She told the story however with great spirit among her friends; for she had a lively, playful disposition, which delighted in any thing ridiculous.

The evening altogether passed off pleasantly to the whole family. Mrs Bennet had seen her eldest daughter much admired by the Netherfield party. Mr Bingley had danced with her twice, and she had been distinguished by his sisters. Jane was as much gratified by this, as her mother could be, though in a quieter way. Elizabeth felt Jane's pleasure. Mary had heard herself mentioned to Miss Bingley as the most accomplished girl in the neighbourhood; and Catherine and Lydia had been fortunate enough to be never without partners, which was all that they had yet learnt to care for at a ball. They returned therefore in good spirits to Longbourn, the village where they lived, and of which they were the principal inhabitants. They found Mr Bennet still up. With a book he was regardless of time; and on the present occasion he had a good deal of curiosity as to the event of an evening which had raised such splendid expectations. He had rather hoped that all his wife's views on the stranger would be disappointed; but he soon found that he had a very different story to hear.

'Oh! my dear Mr Bennet,' as she entered the room, 'we have had a most delightful evening, a most excellent ball. I wish you had been there. Jane was so admired, nothing could be like it. Every body said how well she looked; and Mr Bingley thought her quite beautiful, and danced with her twice. Only think of that my dear; he actually danced with her twice; and she was the only creature in the room that he asked a second time. First of all, he asked Miss Lucas. I was so vexed to see him stand up with her; but, however, he did not admire her at all: indeed, nobody can, you know; and he seemed quite struck with Jane as she was going down the dance. So, he enquired who she was, and got introduced, and asked her for the two next. Then, the two third he danced with Miss King, and the two fourth with Maria Lucas, and the two fifth with Jane again, and the two sixth with Lizzy, and the Boulanger—'

'If he had had any compassion for me,' cried her husband impatiently, 'he would not have danced half so much! For God's sake, say no more of his partners. Oh! that he had sprained his ancle in the first dance!'

'Oh! my dear,' continued Mrs Bennet, 'I am quite delighted with him. He is so excessively handsome! and his sisters are charming women. I never in my life saw any thing more elegant than their dresses. I dare say the lace upon Mrs Hurst's gown—'

Here she was interrupted again. Mr Bennet protested against any description of finery. She was therefore obliged to seek another branch of the subject, and related, with much bitterness of spirit and some exaggeration, the shocking rudeness of Mr Darcy.

'But I can assure you,' she added, 'that Lizzy does not lose much by not suiting *his* fancy; for he is a most disagreeable, horrid man, not at all worth pleasing. So high and so conceited that there was no enduring him! He walked here, and he walked there, fancying himself so very great! Not handsome enough to dance with! I wish you had been there, my dear, to have given him one of your set downs. I quite detest the man.'

ABOUT THE EDITOR

Taesha Glasgow is the creator behind the *Just Sleep* podcast – now ranked as one of the top mental health podcasts with over 20 million downloads. She also works as a consultant helping other podcasters launch and grow their shows. Originally from the Caribbean, she now lives with her husband in Collingham, a village just outside of Leeds.